Skill Checklists to Accompany

Fundamentals of Nursing

THE ART AND SCIENCE OF NURSING CARE

Skill Checklists to Accompany

Fundamentals of Nursing

THE ART AND SCIENCE OF NURSING CARE

SIXTH EDITION

Carol R. Taylor, RN, MSN, PhD
Director, Center for Clinical Bioethics
Assistant Professor of Nursing
Georgetown University
Washington, DC

Carol Lillis, RN, MSN
Faculty Emerita, Assistant to the Provost
Delaware County Community College
Media, Pennsylvania

Priscilla LeMone, RN, DSN, FAAN
Associate Professor Emeritus
Sinclair School of Nursing
University of Missouri-Columbia
Columbia, Missouri

Pamela Lynn, RN, MSN
Faculty
School of Nursing
Gwynedd-Mercy College
Gwynedd Valley, Pennsylvania

Marilee LeBon, BA
Developmental Editor
Mountaintop, PA

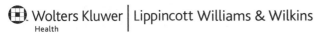 Wolters Kluwer | Lippincott Williams & Wilkins
Health
Philadelphia • Baltimore • New York • London
Buenos Aires • Hong Kong • Sydney • Tokyo

Ancillary Editor: Audrey Lickwar
Senior Production Editor: Sandra Cherrey Scheinin
Director of Nursing Production: Helen Ewan
Senior Managing Editor/Production: Erika Kors
Senior Manufacturing Manager: William Alberti
Compositor: Techbooks
Printer: Victor Graphics

9 8 7 6 5 4

ISBN 13: 978-0-7817-6406-3
ISBN 10: 0-7817-6406-8

Care has been taken to confirm the accuracy of the information presented and to describe generally accepted practices. However, the authors, editors, and publisher are not responsible for errors or omissions or for any consequences from application of the information in this book and make no warranty, express or implied, with respect to the content of the publication.

The authors, editors, and publisher have exerted every effort to ensure that drug selection and dosage set forth in this text are in accordance with the current recommendations and practice at the time of publication. However, in view of ongoing research, changes in government regulations, and the constant flow of information relating to drug therapy and drug reactions, the reader is urged to check the package insert for each drug for any change in indications and dosage and for added warnings and precautions. This is particularly important when the recommended agent is a new or infrequently employed drug.

Some drugs and medical devices presented in this publication have Food and Drug Administration (FDA) clearance for limited use in restricted research settings. It is the responsibility of the health care provider to ascertain the FDA status of each drug or device planned for use in his or her clinical practice.

LWW.com

Introduction

Developing clinical competency is a major challenge for each fundamentals student. To facilitate the mastery of nursing skills, we are happy to provide Skill Checklists for each skill in *Fundamentals of Nursing: The Art and Science of Nursing Care,* 6th edition. The skill checklists follow each step of the skill to provide a complete evaluative tool. Students can use the checklists to facilitate self-evaluation, and faculty will find them useful in measuring and recording student performance. Three-hole-punched and perforated, these checklists can be easily reproduced and brought to the simulation laboratory or clinical area. The checklists are designed to record an evaluation of each step of the skill.

- Checkmark in the "Excellent" column denotes mastering the procedure.
- Checkmark in the "Satisfactory" column indicates use of the recommended technique.
- Checkmark in the "Needs Practice" column indicates use of some but not all of each recommended technique.

The Comments section allows you to highlight suggestions that will improve skills. Space is available at the top of each checklist to record a final pass/fail evaluation, date, and the signature of the student and evaluating faculty member.

List of Skills by Chapter

List of Skills in Alphabetical Order

Skill Checklists to Accompany Fundamentals of Nursing:
The Art and Science of Nursing Care, 6th edition

Name _____ Date _____

Unit _____ Position _____

Instructor/Evaluator: _____ Position _____

Excellent	Satisfactory	Needs Practice	SKILL 24-1 **Assessing Body Temperature**	Comments
			Goal: The patient's temperature is assessed accurately without injury and the patient experiences minimal discomfort.	
____	____	____	1. Check the physician's order or nursing care plan for frequency and route. More frequent temperature measurement may be appropriate based on nursing judgment.	
____	____	____	2. Identify the patient. Discuss procedure with patient and assess the patient's ability to assist with the procedure.	
____	____	____	3. Ensure the electronic or digital thermometer is in working condition.	
____	____	____	4. Close curtains around bed and close door to room if possible.	
____	____	____	5. **Perform hand hygiene and put on gloves if appropriate or indicated.**	
____	____	____	6. Select the appropriate site based on previous assessment data.	
____	____	____	7. Follow the steps as outlined below for the appropriate type of thermometer.	
____	____	____	8. When measurement is completed, remove gloves, if worn. Perform hand hygiene.	
			Measuring a Tympanic Membrane Temperature	
____	____	____	1. If necessary, push the "on" button and wait for the "ready" signal on the unit.	
____	____	____	2. Attach tympanic probe covering.	
____	____	____	3. **Insert the probe snugly into the external ear using gentle but firm pressure, angling the thermometer toward the patient's jaw line. Pull pinna up and back to straighten the ear canal in an adult.**	
____	____	____	4. Activate the unit by pushing the trigger button. The reading is immediate (usually within 2 seconds). Note the reading.	
____	____	____	5. Discard the probe cover in an appropriate receptacle by pushing the probe release button or use rim of cover to remove from probe. Replace the thermometer in its charger, if necessary.	

Excellent	Satisfactory	Needs Practice		Comments

Assessing Oral Temperature

___	___	___	1. Remove the electronic unit from the charging unit, and remove the probe from within the recording unit.
___	___	___	2. Cover thermometer probe with disposable probe cover and slide it on until it snaps into place.
___	___	___	3. **Place the probe beneath the patient's tongue in the posterior sublingual pocket. Ask the patient to close his or her lips around the probe.**
___	___	___	4. **Continue to hold the probe until you hear a beep.** Note the temperature reading.
___	___	___	5. Remove the probe from the patient's mouth. Dispose of the probe cover by holding the probe over an appropriate receptacle and pressing the probe release button.
___	___	___	6. Return the thermometer probe to the storage place within the unit. Return the electronic unit to the charging unit, if appropriate.

Assessing Rectal Temperature

___	___	___	1. Place the bed at an appropriate working height. Put on nonsterile gloves.
___	___	___	2. Assist the patient to a side-lying position. Pull back the covers enough to expose only the buttocks.
___	___	___	3. Remove the rectal probe from within the recording unit of the electronic thermometer. Cover the probe with a disposable probe cover and slide it into place until it snaps in place.
___	___	___	4. **Lubricate about 1″ of the probe with a water-soluble lubricant.**
___	___	___	5. Reassure the patient. Separate the buttocks until the anal sphincter is clearly visible.
___	___	___	6. **Insert the thermometer probe into the anus about 1.5″ in an adult or 1″ in a child.**
___	___	___	7. Hold the probe in place until you hear a beep; then carefully remove the probe. Note the temperature reading on the display.
___	___	___	8. Dispose of the probe cover by holding the probe over an appropriate waste receptacle and pressing the release button.

SKILL 24-1

Assessing Body Temperature *(Continued)*

Excellent	Satisfactory	Needs Practice		Comments
——	——	——	9. Using toilet tissue, wipe the anus of any feces or excess lubricant. Dispose of the toilet tissue.	
——	——	——	10. Cover the patient and help him or her to a position of comfort.	
——	——	——	11. Remove gloves and discard them. Perform hand hygiene.	
——	——	——	12. Place the bed in the lowest position; elevate rails as needed.	
——	——	——	13. Return the thermometer to the charging unit.	
			Assessing Axillary Temperature	
——	——	——	1. Place the bed at an appropriate working height.	
——	——	——	2. Move the patient's clothing to expose only the axilla.	
——	——	——	3. Remove the probe from the recording unit of the electronic thermometer. Place a disposable probe cover on by sliding it on and snapping it securely.	
——	——	——	4. **Place the end of the probe in the center of the axilla. Have the patient bring the arm down and close to the body.**	
——	——	——	5. Hold the probe in place until you hear a beep, and then carefully remove the probe. Note the temperature reading.	
——	——	——	6. Cover the patient and help him or her to a position of comfort.	
——	——	——	7. Dispose of the probe cover by holding the probe over an appropriate waste receptacle and pushing the release button.	
——	——	——	8. Place the bed in the lowest position and elevate rails as needed. Leave the patient clean and comfortable.	
——	——	——	9. Return the electronic thermometer to the charging unit.	

Skill Checklists to Accompany Fundamentals of Nursing:
The Art and Science of Nursing Care, 6th edition

Name _____   Date _____

Unit _____   Position _____

Instructor/Evaluator: _____   Position _____

SKILL 24-2

Assessing a Peripheral Pulse by Palpation

Goal: The patient's pulse is assessed accurately without injury and the patient experiences minimal discomfort.

Excellent	Satisfactory	Needs Practice		Comments
——	——	——	1. Check physician's order or nursing care plan for frequency of pulse assessment. More frequent pulse measurement may be appropriate based on nursing judgment.	
——	——	——	2. Identify the patient.	
——	——	——	3. Explain the procedure to the patient.	
——	——	——	4. Close curtains around bed and close door to room if possible.	
——	——	——	5. Perform hand hygiene and put on gloves as appropriate.	
——	——	——	6. Select the appropriate peripheral site based on assessment data.	
——	——	——	7. Move the patient's clothing to expose only the site chosen.	
——	——	——	8. Place your first, second, and third fingers over the artery. **Lightly compress the artery so pulsations can be felt and counted.**	
——	——	——	9. **Using a watch with a second hand, count the number of pulsations felt for 30 seconds. Multiply this number by 2 to calculate the rate for 1 minute. If the rate, rhythm, or amplitude of the pulse is abnormal in any way, palpate and count the pulse for 1 minute or longer.**	
——	——	——	10. Note the rhythm and amplitude of the pulse.	
——	——	——	11. Cover the patient and help him or her to a position of comfort.	
——	——	——	12. Remove gloves, if necessary. Perform hand hygiene.	

Skill Checklists to Accompany Fundamentals of Nursing:
The Art and Science of Nursing Care, 6th edition

Name _____ Date _____

Unit _____ Position _____

Instructor/Evaluator: _____ Position _____

Excellent	Satisfactory	Needs Practice	SKILL 24-3 **Assessing Respiration**	
			Goal: The patient's respirations are assessed accurately without injury and the patient experiences minimal discomfort.	**Comments**
____	____	____	1. **While your fingers are still in place for the pulse measurement, after counting the pulse rate, observe the patient's respirations.**	
____	____	____	2. Note the rise and fall of the patient's chest.	
____	____	____	3. Using a watch with a second hand, count the number of respirations for 30 seconds. Multiply this number by 2 to calculate the respiratory rate per minute.	
____	____	____	4. If respirations are abnormal in any way, count the respirations for at least 1 full minute.	
____	____	____	5. Note the depth and rhythm of the respirations.	
____	____	____	6. Perform hand hygiene.	

Skill Checklists to Accompany Fundamentals of Nursing:
The Art and Science of Nursing Care, 6th edition

Name _____ Date _____

Unit _____ Position _____

Instructor/Evaluator: _____ Position _____

Excellent	Satisfactory	Needs Practice	SKILL 24-4

SKILL 24-4
Assessing a Brachial Artery Blood Pressure

Goal: The patient's blood pressure is measured accurately without injury.

Comments

Excellent	Satisfactory	Needs Practice		Comments
—	—	—	1. Check physician's order or nursing care plan for frequency of blood pressure measurement. More frequent measurement may be appropriate based on nursing judgment.	
—	—	—	2. Identify the patient.	
—	—	—	3. Explain the procedure to the patient.	
—	—	—	4. Perform hand hygiene and put on gloves if appropriate or indicated.	
—	—	—	5. Close curtains around bed and close door to room if possible.	
—	—	—	6. **Select the appropriate arm for application of cuff.**	
—	—	—	7. Have the patient assume a comfortable lying or sitting position with the forearm supported at the level of the heart and the palm of the hand upward.	
—	—	—	8. Expose the brachial artery by removing garments, or move a sleeve, if it is not too tight, above the area where the cuff will be placed.	
—	—	—	9. **Palpate the location of the brachial artery. Center the bladder of the cuff over the brachial artery, about midway on the arm, so that the lower edge of the cuff is about 2.5 to 5 cm (1″ to 2″) above the inner aspect of the elbow. Line up the artery marking on the cuff with the patient's brachial artery. The tubing should extend from the edge of the cuff nearer the patient's elbow.**	
—	—	—	10. Wrap the cuff around the arm smoothly and snugly, and fasten it. Do not allow any clothing to interfere with the proper placement of the cuff.	
—	—	—	11. Check that the needle on the aneroid gauge is within the zero mark. If using a mercury manometer, check to see that the manometer is in the vertical position and that the mercury is within the zero level with the gauge at eye level.	

SKILL 24-4

Assessing a Brachial Artery Blood Pressure *(Continued)*

Excellent	Satisfactory	Needs Practice		Comments

Estimating Systolic Pressure

____ ____ ____ 12. Palpate the pulse at the brachial or radial artery by pressing gently with the fingertips.

____ ____ ____ 13. Tighten the screw valve on the air pump.

____ ____ ____ 14. Inflate the cuff while continuing to palpate the artery. Note the point on the gauge where the pulse disappears.

____ ____ ____ 15. Deflate the cuff and wait 15 seconds.

Obtaining Blood Pressure Measurement

____ ____ ____ 16. Assume a position that is no more than 3 feet away from the gauge.

____ ____ ____ 17. Place the stethoscope earpieces in your ears. Direct the earpieces forward into the canal and not against the ear itself.

____ ____ ____ 18. Place the bell or diaphragm of the stethoscope firmly but with as little pressure as possible over the brachial artery. Do not allow the stethoscope to touch clothing or the cuff.

____ ____ ____ 19. Pump the pressure 30 mm Hg above the point at which the systolic pressure was palpated and estimated. Open the valve on the manometer and allow air to escape slowly (allowing the gauge to drop 2 to 3 mm per heartbeat).

____ ____ ____ 20. Note the point on the gauge at which the first faint, but clear, sound appears that slowly increases in intensity. Note this number as the systolic pressure.

____ ____ ____ 21. Read the pressure to the closest even number.

____ ____ ____ 22. Do not reinflate the cuff once the air is being released to recheck the systolic pressure reading.

____ ____ ____ 23. Note the pressure at which the sound first becomes muffled. Also observe the point at which the sound completely disappears. These may occur separately or at the same point.

____ ____ ____ 24. Allow the remaining air to escape quickly. Repeat any suspicious reading, but wait 30 to 60 seconds between readings to allow normal circulation to return in the limb. Deflate the cuff completely between attempts to check the blood pressure.

____ ____ ____ 25. Remove the cuff, and clean and store the equipment.

____ ____ ____ 26. Remove gloves, if worn. Perform hand hygiene.

Skill Checklists to Accompany Fundamentals of Nursing:
The Art and Science of Nursing Care, 6th edition

Name _____   Date _____

Unit _____   Position _____

Instructor/Evaluator: _____   Position _____

SKILL 26-1
Applying an Extremity Restraint

Goal: The patient is constrained by the restraint, remains free from injury, and the restraint does not interfere with therapeutic devices.

Excellent	Satisfactory	Needs Practice		Comments
——	——	——	1. Determine need for restraints. Assess patient's physical condition, behavior, and mental status.	
——	——	——	2. Confirm agency policy for application of restraints. **Secure a physician's order, or validate that the order has been obtained within the past 24 hours.**	
——	——	——	3. Identify the patient.	
——	——	——	4. Explain reason for use to patient and family. Clarify how care will be given and how needs will be met. Explain that restraint is a temporary measure.	
——	——	——	5. Perform hand hygiene.	
——	——	——	6. Apply restraint according to manufacturer's directions:	
——	——	——	a. Choose the least restrictive type of device that allows the greatest possible degree of mobility.	
——	——	——	b. Pad bony prominences.	
——	——	——	c. Wrap the restraint around the extremity with the soft part in contact with the skin. If hand mitt is being used, pull over hand with cushion to the palmar aspect of hand. Secure in place with the Velcro straps or reverse clove hitch.	
——	——	——	7. **Ensure that two fingers can be inserted between the restraint and patient's wrist or ankle.**	
——	——	——	8. Maintain restrained extremity in normal anatomic position. **Use a quick-release knot to tie the restraint to the bed frame, not side rail. The restraint may also be attached to chair frame. The site should not be readily accessible to patient.**	

Excellent	Satisfactory	Needs Practice		Comments
——	——	——	9. Assess the patient at least every hour or according to facility policy. Assessment should include: the placement of the restraint, neurovascular assessment of the affected extremity, and skin integrity. In addition, assess for signs of sensory deprivation, such as increased sleeping, daydreaming, anxiety, panic, and hallucinations.	
——	——	——	10. **Remove restraint at least every 2 hours, or according to agency policy and patient need.** Perform range-of-motion exercises.	
——	——	——	11. Evaluate patient for continued need of restraint. Reapply restraint only if continued need is evident and order is still valid.	
——	——	——	12. Reassure patient at regular intervals. Provide continued explanation of rationale for interventions, reorientation if necessary, and plan of care. **Keep call bell within easy reach.**	
——	——	——	13. Perform hand hygiene.	

Skill Checklists to Accompany Fundamentals of Nursing:
The Art and Science of Nursing Care, 6th edition

Name _____ Date _____

Unit _____ Position _____

Instructor/Evaluator: _____ Position _____

Excellent	Satisfactory	Needs Practice	SKILL 27-1 **Performing Hand Hygiene Using Soap and Water (Handwashing)** **Goal:** The hands will be free of visible soiling and transient microorganisms will be eliminated.	Comments
——	——	——	1. Gather the necessary supplies. Stand in front of the sink. Do not allow your clothing to touch the sink during the washing procedure.	
——	——	——	2. Remove jewelry, if possible, and secure in a safe place. A plain wedding band may remain in place.	
——	——	——	3. Turn on water and adjust force. Regulate the temperature until the water is warm.	
——	——	——	4. Wet the hands and wrist area. Keep hands lower than elbows to allow water to flow toward fingertips.	
——	——	——	5. Use about 1 teaspoon liquid soap from dispenser or rinse bar of soap and lather thoroughly. Cover all areas of hands with the soap product. Rinse soap bar again and return to soap dish.	
——	——	——	6. With firm rubbing and circular motions, wash the palms and backs of the hands, each finger, the areas between the fingers, and the knuckles, wrists, and forearms. **Wash at least 1″ above area of contamination.** If hands are not visibly soiled, wash to 1″ above the wrists.	
——	——	——	7. Continue this friction motion for at least 15 seconds.	
——	——	——	8. Use fingernails of the opposite hand or a clean orangewood stick to clean under fingernails.	
——	——	——	9. Rinse thoroughly with water flowing toward fingertips.	
——	——	——	10. Pat hands dry, beginning with the fingers and moving upward toward forearms, with a paper towel and discard it immediately. Use another clean towel to turn off the faucet. Discard towel immediately without touching other clean hand.	
——	——	——	11. Use oil-free lotion on hands if desired.	

Skill Checklists to Accompany Fundamentals of Nursing:
The Art and Science of Nursing Care, 6th edition

Name _____   Date _____

Unit _____   Position _____

Instructor/Evaluator: _____   Position _____

Excellent	Satisfactory	Needs Practice	SKILL 27-2 **Using Personal Protective Equipment**	
			Goal: The transmission of microorganisms is prevented.	**Comments**
___	___	___	1. Check physician's order for type of precautions and review precautions in infection control manual.	
___	___	___	2. Plan nursing activities before entering patient's room.	
___	___	___	3. Provide instruction about precautions to patient, family members, and visitors.	
___	___	___	4. Perform hand hygiene.	
___	___	___	5. Put on gown, gloves, mask, and protective eyewear, based on the type of exposure anticipated and category of isolation precautions.	
___	___	___	a. Put on the gown, with the opening in the back. Tie gown securely at neck and waist.	
___	___	___	b. Put the mask or respirator over your nose, mouth, and chin. Secure ties or elastic bands at the middle of the head and neck. If respirator is used, perform a fit check. Inhale; the respirator should collapse. Exhale; air should not leak out.	
___	___	___	c. Put on goggles. Place over eyes and adjust to fit. Alternately, a face shield could be used to take the place of the mask and goggles.	
___	___	___	d. Put on clean disposable gloves. Extend gloves to cover wrists of gown.	
___	___	___	6. Remove PPE: Except for respirator, remove PPE at the doorway or in anteroom. Remove respirator after leaving the patient room and closing door.	
___	___	___	a. If impervious gown has been tied in front of the body at the waistline, untie waist strings before removing gloves.	
___	___	___	b. Grasp the outside of one glove with the opposite gloved hand and peel off, turning the glove inside out as you pull it off. Hold the removed glove in the remaining gloved hand.	
___	___	___	c. Slide fingers of ungloved hand under the remaining glove at the wrist, taking care not to touch the outer surface of the glove.	

Using Personal Protective Equipment (Continued)

Excellent	Satisfactory	Needs Practice		Comments
——	——	——	d. Peel off the glove over the first glove, containing the one glove inside the other. Discard in appropriate container.	
——	——	——	e. To remove the goggles: Handle by the headband or earpieces. Lift away from the face. Place in designated receptacle for reprocessing or in an appropriate waste container.	
——	——	——	f. To remove gown: Unfasten ties, if at the neck and back. Allow the gown to fall away from shoulders. Touching only the inside of the gown, pull away from the torso. Keeping hands on the inner surface of the gown, pull from arms. Turn gown inside out. Fold or roll into a bundle and discard.	
——	——	——	g. To remove mask or respirator: Grasp the neck ties or elastic, then top ties or elastic and remove. Take care to avoid touching front of mask or respirator. Discard in waste container. If using a respirator, save for future use in the designated area.	
——	——	——	7. Perform hand hygiene immediately after removing all PPE.	

Skill Checklists to Accompany Fundamentals of Nursing:
The Art and Science of Nursing Care, 6th edition

Name _____   Date _____

Unit _____   Position _____

Instructor/Evaluator: _____   Position _____

Excellent	Satisfactory	Needs Practice	SKILL 27-3 **Preparing a Sterile Field Using a Packaged Sterile Drape**	Comments
			Goal: The sterile field is created without evidence of contamination and the patient remains free of exposure to potential infection-causing microorganisms.	
⎯	⎯	⎯	1. Identify the patient. Explain the procedure to the patient.	
⎯	⎯	⎯	2. Perform hand hygiene.	
			Preparing a Sterile Field	
⎯	⎯	⎯	3. Check that packaged sterile drape or tray is dry and unopened. Also note expiration date, making sure that the date is still valid.	
⎯	⎯	⎯	4. Select a work area that is waist level or higher.	
⎯	⎯	⎯	5. Open sterile wrapped drape or commercially prepared kit. For a prepackaged sterile drape:	
⎯	⎯	⎯	a. Open the outer covering of the drape. Remove sterile drape, lifting it carefully by its corners. Hold away from body and above the waist and work surface.	
⎯	⎯	⎯	b. Continue to hold only by the corners. Allow the drape to unfold, away from your body and any other surface.	
⎯	⎯	⎯	c. Position the drape on the work surface with the moisture-proof side down. This would be the shiny or blue side. Avoid touching any other surface or object with the drape.	
			For a commercially prepared kit or tray:	
⎯	⎯	⎯	a. Open the outside cover of the package and remove the kit or tray. Place in the center of the work surface.	
⎯	⎯	⎯	b. Reach around the package and grasp the outer surface of the end of the topmost flap, holding no more than 1 inch from the border of the flap. Pull open away from the body, keeping the arm outstretched and away from the inside of the wrapper. Allow the wrapper to lie flat on the work surface.	
⎯	⎯	⎯	c. Reach around the package and grasp the outer surface of the first side flap, holding no more than 1 inch from the border of the flap. Pull open to the side of the package, keeping the arm outstretched and away from the inside of the wrapper. Allow the wrapper to lie flat on the work surface.	

SKILL 27-3
Preparing a Sterile Field Using a Packaged Sterile Drape *(Continued)*

Excellent	Satisfactory	Needs Practice		Comments

   —— —— —— d. Reach around the package and grasp the outer surface of the remaining side flap, holding no more than 1 inch from the border of the flap. Pull open to the side of the package, keeping the arm outstretched and away from the inside of the wrapper. Allow the wrapper to lie flat on the work surface.

   —— —— —— e. Stand away from the package and work surface. Grasp the outer surface of the remaining flap closest to the body, holding no more than 1 inch from the border of the flap. Pull the flap back toward the body, keeping arm outstretched and away from the inside of the wrapper. Allow the wrapper to lie flat on the work surface.

   —— —— —— f. The outer wrapper of the package has become a sterile field with the package's supplies in the center. Do not touch or reach over the sterile field.

Adding Items to a Sterile Field

   —— —— —— 6. Add sterile item.
To add an agency-wrapped and sterilized item:

   —— —— —— a. Hold agency-wrapped item in the dominant hand with top flap opening away from the body. With other hand, reach around the package and unfold top flap and both sides.

   —— —— —— b. Keep a secure hold on item through the wrapper with the dominant hand. Grasp the remaining flap of the wrapper closet to the body, taking care not to touch the inner surface of the wrapper or the item. Pull the flap back toward the wrist, so the wrapper covers the hand and wrist.

   —— —— —— c. Grasp all the corners of the wrapper together with the nondominant hand and pull back toward wrist, covering hand and wrist. Hold in place.

   —— —— —— d. Hold the item 6 inches above the surface of the sterile field and drop onto the field. Be careful to avoid touching the surface or other items or dropping onto the 1-inch border.

To add a commercially wrapped and sterilized item:

   —— —— —— a. Hold package in one hand. Pull back top cover with other hand. Alternately, carefully peel the edges apart using both hands.

Preparing a Sterile Field Using a Packaged Sterile Drape *(Continued)*

Excellent	Satisfactory	Needs Practice		Comments

b. After top cover or edges are partially separated, hold the item 6 inches above the surface of the sterile field. Continue opening the package and drop the item onto the field. Be careful to avoid touching the surface or other items or dropping onto the 1-inch border.

c. Discard wrapper.

To add a sterile solution:

a. Obtain appropriate solution and check expiration date.

b. Open solution container according to directions and place cap on table with edges up.

c. If bottle has previously been opened, "lip" it by pouring a small amount of solution into waste container.

d. Hold bottle outside the edge of the sterile field with the label side facing the palm of your hand and prepare to pour from a height of 4 to 6 inches (10 to 15 cm). The tip of the bottle should never touch a sterile container or dressing.

e. Pour required amount of solution steadily into sterile container positioned at side of sterile field or onto dressings. Avoid splashing any liquid.

f. Touch only the outside of the lid when recapping. Label solution with date and time of opening.

7. Continue with procedure as indicated.

Skill Checklists to Accompany Fundamentals of Nursing:
The Art and Science of Nursing Care, 6th edition

Name _____ Date _____

Unit _____ Position _____

Instructor/Evaluator: _____ Position _____

SKILL 27-4

Putting on Sterile Gloves and Removing Soiled Gloves

Goal: The gloves are applied and removed without contamination.

Excellent	Satisfactory	Needs Practice		Comments
——	——	——	1. Identify the patient. Explain the procedure to the patient.	
——	——	——	2. Perform hand hygiene.	
——	——	——	3. Check that the sterile glove package is dry and unopened. Also note expiration date, making sure that the date is still valid.	
——	——	——	4. Place sterile glove package on clean, dry surface at or above your waist.	
——	——	——	5. Open the outside wrapper by carefully peeling the top layer back. Remove inner package, handling only the outside of it.	
——	——	——	6. Place the inner package on the work surface with the side labeled "cuff end" closest to the body.	
——	——	——	7. Carefully open the inner package. Fold open the top flap, then the bottom and sides. Take care not to touch the inner surface of the package or the gloves.	
——	——	——	8. With the thumb and forefinger of the nondominant hand, grasp the folded cuff of the glove for dominant hand, touching only the exposed inside of the glove.	
——	——	——	9. Keeping the hands above the waistline, lift and hold the glove up and off the inner package with fingers down. **Be careful it does not touch any unsterile object.**	
——	——	——	10. Carefully insert dominant hand palm up into glove and pull glove on. Leave the cuff folded until the opposite hand is gloved.	
——	——	——	11. Hold the thumb of the gloved hand outward. Place the fingers of the gloved hand inside the cuff of the remaining glove. Lift it from the wrapper, taking care not to touch anything with the gloves or hands.	
——	——	——	12. Carefully insert nondominant hand into glove. Pull the glove on, taking care that the skin does not touch any of the outer surfaces of the gloves.	

SKILL 27-4

Putting on Sterile Gloves and Removing Soiled Gloves *(Continued)*

Excellent	Satisfactory	Needs Practice		Comments
____	____	____	13. Slide the fingers of one hand under the cuff of the other and fully extend the cuff down the arm, touching only the sterile outside of the glove. Repeat for the remaining hand.	
____	____	____	14. **Adjust gloves on both hands if necessary, touching only sterile areas with other sterile areas.**	
____	____	____	15. Continue with procedure as indicated.	
			Removing Soiled Gloves	
____	____	____	16. Use dominant hand to grasp the opposite glove near cuff end on the outside exposed area. Remove it by pulling it off, inverting it as it is pulled, keeping the contaminated area on the inside. Hold the removed glove in the remaining gloved hand.	
____	____	____	17. Slide fingers of ungloved hand between the remaining glove and the wrist. Take care to avoid touching the outside surface of the glove. Remove it by pulling it off, inverting it as it is pulled, keeping the contaminated area on the inside, and securing the first glove inside the second.	
____	____	____	18. Discard gloves in appropriate container and perform hand hygiene.	

Skill Checklists to Accompany Fundamentals of Nursing:
The Art and Science of Nursing Care, 6th edition

Name _____   Date _____

Unit _____   Position _____

Instructor/Evaluator: _____   Position _____

SKILL 29-1
Administering Oral Medications

Goal: The patient will swallow the medication.

Excellent	Satisfactory	Needs Practice		Comments
⎯⎯	⎯⎯	⎯⎯	1. Gather equipment. Check each medication order against the original physician's order according to agency policy. Clarify any inconsistencies. Check the patient's chart for allergies.	
⎯⎯	⎯⎯	⎯⎯	2. Know the actions, special nursing considerations, safe dose ranges, purpose of administration, and adverse effects of the medications to be administered. Consider the appropriateness of the medication for this patient.	
⎯⎯	⎯⎯	⎯⎯	3. Perform hand hygiene.	
⎯⎯	⎯⎯	⎯⎯	4. Move the medication cart to the outside of the patient's room or prepare for administration in the medication area.	
⎯⎯	⎯⎯	⎯⎯	5. Unlock the medication cart or drawer. Enter pass code and scan employee identification, if required.	
⎯⎯	⎯⎯	⎯⎯	6. **Prepare medications for one patient at a time.**	
⎯⎯	⎯⎯	⎯⎯	7. Read the MAR and select the proper medication from the patient's medication drawer or unit stock.	
⎯⎯	⎯⎯	⎯⎯	8. Compare the label with the MAR. Check expiration dates and perform calculations, if necessary. Scan the barcode on the package, if required.	
⎯⎯	⎯⎯	⎯⎯	9. Prepare the required medications:	
⎯⎯	⎯⎯	⎯⎯	a. *Unit dose packages:* Place unit dose-packaged medications in a disposable cup. **Do not open wrapper until at the bedside.** Keep narcotics and medications that require special nursing assessments in a separate container.	
⎯⎯	⎯⎯	⎯⎯	b. *Multidose containers:* When removing tablets or capsules from a multidose bottle, pour the necessary number into the bottle cap and then place the tablets in a medication cup. Break only scored tablets, if necessary, to obtain the proper dosage. Do not touch tablets with hands.	

Excellent	Satisfactory	Needs Practice	SKILL 29-1 **Administering Oral Medications** *(Continued)*	Comments
——	——	——	c. *Liquid medication in multidose bottle:* When pouring liquid medications in a multidose bottle, hold the bottle so the label is against the palm. Use the appropriate measuring device when pouring liquids, and read the amount of medication at the bottom of the meniscus at eye level. Wipe the lip of the bottle with a paper towel.	
——	——	——	10. **When all medications for one patient have been prepared, recheck the label with the MAR before taking them to the patient. Replace any multidose containers in the patient's drawer or unit stock. Lock the medication cart before leaving it.**	
——	——	——	11. Transport medications to the patient's bedside carefully, and keep the medications in sight at all times.	
——	——	——	12. **Ensure that the patient receives the medications at the correct time.**	
——	——	——	13. **Identify the patient.** Usually, the patient should be identified using two methods. Compare information with the MAR or CMAR.	
——	——	——	a. Check the name and identification number on the patient's identification band.	
——	——	——	b. Ask the patient to state his or her name.	
——	——	——	c. If the patient cannot identify him or herself, verify the patient's identification with a staff member who knows the patient for the second source.	
——	——	——	14. **Complete necessary assessments before administering medications. Check allergy bracelet or ask patient about allergies. Explain the purpose and action of each medication to the patient.**	
——	——	——	15. Scan the patient's barcode on the identification band, if required.	
——	——	——	16. Assist the patient to an upright or lateral position.	
——	——	——	17. Administer medications:	
——	——	——	a. Offer water or other permitted fluids with pills, capsules, tablets, and some liquid medications.	
——	——	——	b. Ask whether the patient prefers to take the medications by hand or in a cup.	

Excellent	Satisfactory	Needs Practice		Comments
			SKILL 29-1 **Administering Oral Medications** *(Continued)*	
——	——	——	18. **Remain with the patient until each medication is swallowed. Never leave medication at the patient's bedside.** Record the medication administration.	
——	——	——	19. Perform hand hygiene. Leave the patient in a comfortable position.	
——	——	——	20. Check on the patient within 30 minutes, or time appropriate for drug(s), to verify response to medication.	

Skill Checklists to Accompany Fundamentals of Nursing:
The Art and Science of Nursing Care, 6th edition

Name _____   Date _____

Unit _____   Position _____

Instructor/Evaluator: _____   Position _____

Excellent	Satisfactory	Needs Practice	SKILL 29-2 **Removing Medication From an Ampule**	Comments
			Goal: The medication will be removed in a sterile manner, be free from glass shards, and be prepared in the proper dose.	
____	____	____	1. Gather equipment. Check the medication order against the original physician's order according to agency policy. Clarify any inconsistencies. Check the patient's chart for allergies.	
____	____	____	2. Know the actions, special nursing considerations, safe dose ranges, purpose of administration, and adverse effects of the medications to be administered. Consider the appropriateness of the medication for this patient.	
____	____	____	3. Perform hand hygiene.	
____	____	____	4. Move the medication cart to the outside of the patient's room or prepare for administration in the medication area.	
____	____	____	5. Unlock the medication cart or drawer. Enter pass code and scan employee identification, if required.	
____	____	____	6. **Prepare medications for one patient at a time.**	
____	____	____	7. Read the MAR and select the proper medication from the patient's medication drawer or unit stock.	
____	____	____	8. Compare the label with the MAR. Check expiration dates and perform calculations, if necessary. Scan the barcode on the package, if required.	
____	____	____	9. Tap the stem of the ampule or twist your wrist quickly while holding the ampule vertically.	
____	____	____	10. **Wrap a small gauze pad around the neck of the ampule.**	
____	____	____	11. Use a snapping motion to break off the top of the ampule along the scored line at its neck. Always break away from your body.	
____	____	____	12. Attach filter needle to syringe. **Remove the cap from the filter needle by pulling it straight off. Insert the filter needle into the ampule, being careful not to touch the rim.**	
____	____	____	13. Withdraw medication in the amount ordered plus a small amount more (approximately 30%). **Do not inject air into the solution.** Use either of the following methods:	

Excellent	Satisfactory	Needs Practice	SKILL 29-2 **Removing Medication From an Ampule** *(Continued)*	Comments
——	——	——	a. Insert the tip of the needle into the ampule, which is upright on a flat surface, and withdraw fluid into the syringe. **Touch plunger at knob only.**	
——	——	——	b. Insert the tip of the needle into the ampule and invert the ampule. Keep the needle centered and not touching the sides of the ampule. Withdraw fluid into syringe. **Touch plunger at knob only.**	
——	——	——	14. **Wait until the needle has been withdrawn to tap the syringe and expel the air carefully by pushing on the plunger. Check the amount of medication in the syringe with the medication dose and discard any surplus according to facility policy.**	
——	——	——	15. **Recheck the label with the MAR.**	
——	——	——	16. Engage safety guard on filter needle and remove. Discard the filter needle in a suitable container. Attach appropriate administration device to syringe.	
——	——	——	17. Discard the ampule in a suitable container.	
——	——	——	18. Lock the medication cart before leaving it.	
——	——	——	19. Perform hand hygiene.	
——	——	——	20. Proceed with administration, based on prescribed route.	

Skill Checklists to Accompany Fundamentals of Nursing:
The Art and Science of Nursing Care, 6th edition

Name _____   Date _____

Unit _____   Position _____

Instructor/Evaluator: _____   Position _____

Excellent	Satisfactory	Needs Practice	SKILL 29-3 **Removing Medication From a Vial**	Comments
			Goal: Withdrawal of the medication into a syringe in a sterile manner with the proper dose prepared.	
____	____	____	1. Gather equipment. Check the medication order against the original physician's order according to agency policy.	
____	____	____	2. Know the actions, special nursing considerations, safe dose ranges, purpose of administration, and adverse effects of the medications to be administered. Consider the appropriateness of the medication for this patient.	
____	____	____	3. Perform hand hygiene.	
____	____	____	4. Move the medication cart to the outside of the patient's room or prepare for administration in the medication area.	
____	____	____	5. Unlock the medication cart or drawer. Enter pass code and scan employee identification, if required.	
____	____	____	6. **Prepare medications for one patient at a time.**	
____	____	____	7. Read the MAR and select the proper medication from the patient's medication drawer or unit stock.	
____	____	____	8. Compare the label with the MAR. Check expiration dates and perform calculations, if necessary. Scan the barcode on the package, if required.	
____	____	____	9. Remove the metal or plastic cap on the vial that protects the rubber stopper.	
____	____	____	10. **Swab the rubber top with the antimicrobial swab and allow to dry.**	
____	____	____	11. Remove the cap from the needle or blunt cannula by pulling it straight off. Touch the plunger at the knob only. Draw back an amount of air into the syringe that is equal to the specific dose of medication to be withdrawn. Some agencies recommend use of a filter needle when withdrawing premixed medication from multidose vials.	
____	____	____	12. Hold the vial on a flat surface. Pierce the rubber stopper in the center with the needle tip and inject the measured air into the space above the solution. Do not inject air into the solution.	
____	____	____	13. **Invert the vial. Keep the tip of the needle or blunt cannula below the fluid level.**	

24

Removing Medication From a Vial *(Continued)*

Excellent	Satisfactory	Needs Practice		Comments
——	——	——	14. Hold the vial in one hand and use the other to withdraw the medication. Touch the plunger at the knob only. **Draw up the prescribed amount of medication while holding the syringe vertically and at eye level.**	
——	——	——	15. If any air bubbles accumulate in the syringe, tap the barrel of the syringe sharply and move the needle past the fluid into the air space to reinject the air bubble into the vial. Return the needle tip to the solution and continue withdrawal of the medication.	
——	——	——	16. After the correct dose is withdrawn, remove the needle from the vial and carefully replace the cap over the needle. If a filter needle has been used to draw up the medication, remove it and attach the appropriate administration device. Some agencies recommend changing the needle, if one was used to withdraw the medication, before administering the medication.	
——	——	——	17. **Check the amount of medication in the syringe with the medication dose and discard any surplus.**	
——	——	——	18. **Recheck the label with the MAR.**	
——	——	——	19. **If a multidose vial is being used, label the vial with the date and time opened, and store the vial containing the remaining medication according to agency policy.**	
——	——	——	20. Lock the medication cart before leaving it.	
——	——	——	21. Perform hand hygiene.	
——	——	——	22. Proceed with administration, based on prescribed route.	

Skill Checklists to Accompany Fundamentals of Nursing:
The Art and Science of Nursing Care, 6th edition

Name _____   Date _____

Unit _____   Position _____

Instructor/Evaluator: _____   Position _____

Excellent	Satisfactory	Needs Practice	SKILL 29-4 **Mixing Medications From Two Vials in One Syringe**	Comments
			Goal: The accurate withdrawal of the medication into a syringe in a sterile manner with the proper dose prepared.	
____	____	____	1. Gather equipment. Check medication order against the original physician's order according to agency policy.	
____	____	____	2. Know the actions, special nursing considerations, safe dose ranges, purpose of administration, and adverse effects of the medications to be administered. Consider the appropriateness of the medication for this patient.	
____	____	____	3. Perform hand hygiene.	
____	____	____	4. Move the medication cart to the outside of the patient's room or prepare for administration in the medication area.	
____	____	____	5. Unlock the medication cart or drawer. Enter pass code and scan employee identification, if required.	
____	____	____	6. **Prepare medications for one patient at a time.**	
____	____	____	7. Read the MAR and select the proper medications from the patient's medication drawer or unit stock.	
____	____	____	8. Compare the labels with the MAR. Check expiration dates and perform calculations, if necessary. Scan the barcode on the package, if required.	
____	____	____	9. If necessary, remove the cap that protects the rubber stopper on each vial.	
____	____	____	10. **If insulin is a suspension (eg, NPH, Lente), roll and agitate the vial to mix it well.**	
____	____	____	11. Cleanse the rubber tops with antimicrobial swabs.	
____	____	____	12. Remove cap from needle by pulling it straight off. Touch the plunger at the knob only. Draw back an amount of air into the syringe that is equal to the dose of modified insulin to be withdrawn.	
____	____	____	13. Hold the modified vial on a flat surface. Pierce the rubber stopper in the center with the needle tip and inject the measured air into the space above the solution. Do not inject air into the solution. Withdraw the needle.	
____	____	____	14. Draw back an amount of air into the syringe that is equal to the dose of unmodified insulin to be withdrawn.	

Excellent	Satisfactory	Needs Practice		Comments
			SKILL 29-4 **Mixing Medications From Two Vials in One Syringe** *(Continued)*	

Excellent	Satisfactory	Needs Practice		Comments
——	——	——	15. Hold the unmodified vial on a flat surface. Pierce the rubber stopper in the center with the needle tip and inject the measured air into the space above the solution. Do not inject air into the solution. Keep the needle in the vial.	
——	——	——	16. Invert vial of unmodified insulin. Hold the vial in one hand and use the other to withdraw the medication. Touch the plunger at the knob only. **Draw up the prescribed amount of medication while holding the syringe at eye level and vertically.** Turn the vial over and then remove needle from vial.	
——	——	——	17. Check that there are no air bubbles in the syringe.	
——	——	——	18. **Check the amount of medication in the syringe with the medication dose and discard any surplus.**	
——	——	——	19. **Recheck the vial label with the MAR.**	
——	——	——	20. Calculate the endpoint on the syringe for the combined insulin amount by adding the number of units for each dose together.	
——	——	——	21. Insert the needle into the modified vial and invert it, taking care not to push the plunger and inject medication from the syringe into the vial. Invert vial of modified insulin. Hold the vial in one hand and use the other to withdraw the medication. Touch the plunger at the knob only. **Draw up the prescribed amount of medication while holding the syringe at eye level and vertically. Take care to withdraw only the prescribed amount.** Turn the vial over and then remove needle from vial. Carefully recap the needle. Carefully replace the cap over the needle.	
——	——	——	22. **Check the amount of medication in the syringe with the medication dose.**	
——	——	——	23. **Recheck the vial label with the MAR.**	
——	——	——	24. **Label the vials with the date and time opened, and store the vials containing the remaining medication according to agency policy.**	
——	——	——	25. Lock medication cart before leaving it.	
——	——	——	26. Perform hand hygiene.	
——	——	——	27. Proceed with administration, based on prescribed route.	

Skill Checklists to Accompany Fundamentals of Nursing:
The Art and Science of Nursing Care, 6th edition

Name _____ Date _____

Unit _____ Position _____

Instructor/Evaluator: _____ Position _____

Excellent	Satisfactory	Needs Practice	SKILL 29-5 **Administering an Intradermal Injection**	
			Goal: Appearance of a wheal at the site of injection.	**Comments**
____	____	____	1. Gather equipment. Check each medication order against the original physician's order according to agency policy. Clarify any inconsistencies. Check the patient's chart for allergies.	
____	____	____	2. Know the actions, special nursing considerations, safe dose ranges, purpose of administration, and adverse effects of the medications to be administered. Consider the appropriateness of the medication for this patient.	
____	____	____	3. Perform hand hygiene.	
____	____	____	4. Move the medication cart to the outside of the patient's room or prepare for administration in the medication area.	
____	____	____	5. Unlock the medication cart or drawer. Enter pass code and scan employee identification, if required.	
____	____	____	6. **Prepare medications for one patient at a time.**	
____	____	____	7. Read the MAR and select the proper medication from the patient's medication drawer or unit stock.	
____	____	____	8. Compare the label with the MAR. Check expiration dates and perform calculations, if necessary. Scan the barcode on the package, if required.	
____	____	____	9. If necessary, withdraw medication from an ampule or vial as described in Skills 29-2 and 29-3.	
____	____	____	10. **When all medications for one patient have been prepared, recheck the label with the MAR before taking them to the patient.**	
____	____	____	11. Lock the medication cart before leaving it.	
____	____	____	12. Transport medications to the patient's bedside carefully, and keep the medications in sight at all times.	
____	____	____	13. **Ensure that the patient receives the medications at the correct time.**	
____	____	____	14. **Identify the patient.** Usually, the patient should be identified using two methods. Compare information with the MAR or CMAR.	

SKILL 29-5
Administering an Intradermal Injection *(Continued)*

Excellent	Satisfactory	Needs Practice		Comments
—	—	—	a. Check the name and identification number on the patient's identification band.	
—	—	—	b. Ask the patient to state his or her name.	
—	—	—	c. If the patient cannot identify him or herself, verify the patient's identification with a staff member who knows the patient for the second source.	
—	—	—	15. Close the door to the room or pull the bedside curtain.	
—	—	—	16. Complete necessary assessments before administering medications. Check allergy bracelet or ask patient about allergies. Explain the purpose and action of the medication to the patient.	
—	—	—	17. Scan the patient's barcode on the identification band, if required.	
—	—	—	18. Perform hand hygiene and put on clean gloves.	
—	—	—	19. Select an appropriate administration site. Assist the patient to the appropriate position for the site chosen. Drape as needed to expose only area of site to be used.	
—	—	—	20. Cleanse the site with an antimicrobial swab while wiping with a firm, circular motion and moving outward from the injection site. Allow the skin to dry.	
—	—	—	21. Remove the needle cap with the nondominant hand by pulling it straight off.	
—	—	—	22. Use the nondominant hand to spread the skin taut over the injection site.	
—	—	—	23. Hold the syringe in the dominant hand, between the thumb and forefinger with the bevel of the needle up.	
—	—	—	24. Hold the syringe at a 10- to 15-degree angle from the site. **Place the needle almost flat against the patient's skin, bevel side up, and insert the needle into the skin so that the point of the needle can be seen through the skin. Insert the needle only about 1/8″ with entire bevel under the skin.**	
—	—	—	25. Once the needle is in place, steady the lower end of the syringe, and slide your dominant hand to the end of the plunger.	
—	—	—	26. Slowly inject the agent while watching for a small wheal or blister to appear.	
—	—	—	27. Withdraw the needle quickly at the same angle that it was inserted.	

SKILL 29-5

Administering an Intradermal Injection *(Continued)*

Excellent	Satisfactory	Needs Practice		Comments
——	——	——	28. Do not massage area after removing needle. Tell the patient not to rub or scratch the site. If necessary, gently blot the site with a dry gauze square. Do not apply pressure or rub the site.	
——	——	——	29. Do not recap the used needle. Engage the safety shield or needle guard, if present. Discard the needle and syringe in the appropriate receptacle.	
——	——	——	30. Assist the patient to a position of comfort.	
——	——	——	31. Remove gloves and dispose of them properly. Perform hand hygiene.	
——	——	——	32. Observe the area for signs of a reaction at determined intervals after administration. Inform the patient of the need for inspection.	

Skill Checklists to Accompany Fundamentals of Nursing:
The Art and Science of Nursing Care, 6th edition

Name _____ Date _____

Unit _____ Position _____

Instructor/Evaluator: _____ Position _____

SKILL 29-6
Administering a Subcutaneous Injection

Goal: The patient receives medication via the subcutaneous route.

Excellent	Satisfactory	Needs Practice		Comments
——	——	——	1. Gather equipment. Check each medication order against the original physician's order according to agency policy. Clarify any inconsistencies. Check the patient's chart for allergies.	
——	——	——	2. Know the actions, special nursing considerations, safe dose ranges, purpose of administration, and adverse effects of the medications to be administered. Consider the appropriateness of the medication for this patient.	
——	——	——	3. Perform hand hygiene.	
——	——	——	4. Move the medication cart to the outside of the patient's room or prepare for administration in the medication area.	
——	——	——	5. Unlock the medication cart or drawer. Enter pass code and scan employee identification, if required.	
——	——	——	6. **Prepare medications for one patient at a time.**	
——	——	——	7. Read the MAR and select the proper medication from the patient's medication drawer or unit stock.	
——	——	——	8. Compare the label with the MAR. Check expiration dates and perform calculations, if necessary. Scan the barcode on the package, if required.	
——	——	——	9. If necessary, withdraw medication from an ampule or vial as described in Skills 29-2 and 29-3.	
——	——	——	10. **When all medications for one patient have been prepared, recheck the label with the MAR before taking them to the patient.**	
——	——	——	11. Lock the medication cart before leaving it.	
——	——	——	12. Transport medications to the patient's bedside carefully, and keep the medications in sight at all times.	
——	——	——	13. **Ensure that the patient receives the medications at the correct time.**	
——	——	——	14. **Identify the patient.** Usually, the patient should be identified using two methods. Compare information with the MAR or CMAR.	

Excellent	Satisfactory	Needs Practice	SKILL 29-6 **Administering a Subcutaneous Injection** *(Continued)*	
				Comments
——	——	——	a. Check the name and identification number on the patient's identification band.	
——	——	——	b. Ask the patient to state his or her name.	
——	——	——	c. If the patient cannot identify him or herself, verify the patient's identification with a staff member who knows the patient for the second source.	
——	——	——	15. Close the door to the room or pull the bedside curtain.	
——	——	——	16. Complete necessary assessments before administering medications. Check allergy bracelet or ask patient about allergies. Explain the purpose and action of the medication to the patient.	
——	——	——	17. Scan the patient's barcode on the identification band, if required.	
——	——	——	18. Perform hand hygiene and put on clean gloves.	
——	——	——	19. Select an appropriate administration site.	
——	——	——	20. Assist the patient to the appropriate position for the site chosen. Drape as needed to expose only area of site to be used.	
——	——	——	21. Identify the appropriate landmarks for the site chosen.	
——	——	——	22. Clean the area around the injection site with an antimicrobial swab. Use a firm, circular motion while moving outward from the injection site. Allow area to dry.	
——	——	——	23. Remove the needle cap with the nondominant hand, pulling it straight off.	
——	——	——	24. Grasp and bunch the area surrounding the injection site or spread the skin taut at the site.	
——	——	——	25. **Hold the syringe in the dominant hand between the thumb and forefinger. Inject the needle quickly at a 45- to 90-degree angle.**	
——	——	——	26. After the needle is in place, release the tissue. If you have a large skin fold pinched up, ensure that the needle stays in place as the skin is released. Immediately move your nondominant hand to steady the lower end of the syringe. Slide your dominant hand to the end of the plunger. Avoid moving the syringe.	
——	——	——	27. Inject the medication slowly (at a rate of 10 seconds per milliliter).	
——	——	——	28. Withdraw the needle quickly at the same angle at which it was inserted, while supporting the surrounding tissue with your nondominant hand.	

SKILL 29-6
Administering a Subcutaneous Injection *(Continued)*

Excellent	Satisfactory	Needs Practice		Comments
——	——	——	29. Using a gauze square, apply gentle pressure to the site after the needle is withdrawn. Do not massage the site.	
——	——	——	30. Do not recap the used needle. Engage the safety shield or needle guard, if present. Discard the needle and syringe in the appropriate receptacle.	
——	——	——	31. Assist the patient to a position of comfort.	
——	——	——	32. Remove gloves and dispose of them properly. Perform hand hygiene.	
——	——	——	33. Evaluate the response of the patient to the medication within an appropriate time frame for the particular medication.	

Skill Checklists to Accompany Fundamentals of Nursing:
The Art and Science of Nursing Care, 6th edition

Name _____ Date _____

Unit _____ Position _____

Instructor/Evaluator: _____ Position _____

SKILL 29-7
Administering an Intramuscular Injection

Goal: The patient receives the medication via the intramuscular route.

Excellent	Satisfactory	Needs Practice		Comments
___	___	___	1. Gather equipment. Check each medication order against the original physician's order according to agency policy. Clarify any inconsistencies. Check the patient's chart for allergies.	
___	___	___	2. Know the actions, special nursing considerations, safe dose ranges, purpose of administration, and adverse effects of the medications to be administered. Consider the appropriateness of the medication for this patient.	
___	___	___	3. Perform hand hygiene.	
___	___	___	4. Move the medication cart to the outside of the patient's room or prepare for administration in the medication area.	
___	___	___	5. Unlock the medication cart or drawer. Enter pass code and scan employee identification, if required.	
___	___	___	6. **Prepare medications for one patient at a time.**	
___	___	___	7. Read the MAR and select the proper medication from the patient's medication drawer or unit stock.	
___	___	___	8. Compare the label with the MAR. Check expiration dates and perform calculations, if necessary. Scan the barcode on the package, if required.	
___	___	___	9. If necessary, withdraw medication from an ampule or vial as described in Skills 29-2 and 29-3.	
___	___	___	10. **When all medications for one patient have been prepared, recheck the label with the MAR before taking them to the patient.**	
___	___	___	11. Lock the medication cart before leaving it.	
___	___	___	12. Transport medications to the patient's bedside carefully, and keep the medications in sight at all times.	
___	___	___	13. **Ensure that the patient receives the medications at the correct time.**	
___	___	___	14. **Identify the patient.** Usually, the patient should be identified using two methods. Compare information with the MAR or CMAR.	

Excellent	Satisfactory	Needs Practice	SKILL 29-7 **Administering an Intramuscular Injection** *(Continued)*	Comments
——	——	——	a. Check the name and identification number on the patient's identification band.	
——	——	——	b. Ask the patient to state his or her name.	
——	——	——	c. If the patient cannot identify him or herself, verify the patient's identification with a staff member who knows the patient for the second source.	
——	——	——	15. Close the door to the room or pull the bedside curtain.	
——	——	——	16. Complete necessary assessments before administering medications. Check allergy bracelet or ask patient about allergies. Explain the purpose and action of the medication to the patient.	
——	——	——	17. Scan the patient's barcode on the identification band, if required.	
——	——	——	18. Perform hand hygiene and put on clean gloves.	
——	——	——	19. Select an appropriate administration site.	
——	——	——	20. Assist the patient to the appropriate position for the site chosen. Drape as needed to expose only area of site to be used.	
——	——	——	21. **Identify the appropriate landmarks for the site chosen.**	
——	——	——	22. Clean the area around the injection site with an antimicrobial swab. Use a firm, circular motion while moving outward from the injection site. Allow area to dry.	
——	——	——	23. Remove the needle cap by pulling it straight off. Hold the syringe in your dominant hand between the thumb and forefinger.	
——	——	——	24. Displace the skin in a Z-track manner by pulling the skin down or to one side about 1″ (2.5 cm) with your nondominant hand and hold the skin and tissue in this position.	
——	——	——	25. Quickly dart the needle into the tissue so that the needle is perpendicular to the patient's body. This should ensure that it is given using an angle of injection between 72 and 90 degrees.	
——	——	——	26. As soon as the needle is in place, use your thumb and forefinger of your nondominant hand to hold the lower end of the syringe. Slide your dominant hand to the end of the plunger.	
——	——	——	27. **Aspirate by slowly (for at least 5 seconds) pulling back on the plunger to determine whether the needle is in a blood vessel. Watch for a flash of pink or red in the syringe.**	

SKILL 29-7
Administering an Intramuscular Injection *(Continued)*

Excellent	Satisfactory	Needs Practice		Comments
——	——	——	28. If no blood is aspirated, inject the solution slowly (10 seconds per milliliter of medication).	
——	——	——	29. Once the medication has been instilled, wait 10 seconds before withdrawing the needle.	
——	——	——	30. Withdraw the needle smoothly and steadily at the same angle at which it was inserted, supporting tissue around the injection site with your nondominant hand.	
——	——	——	31. **Apply gentle pressure at the site with a dry gauze.**	
——	——	——	32. Do not recap the used needle. Engage the safety shield or needle guard, if present. Discard the needle and syringe in the appropriate receptacle.	
——	——	——	33. Assist the patient to a position of comfort.	
——	——	——	34. Remove gloves and dispose of them properly. Perform hand hygiene.	
——	——	——	35. Evaluate patient's response to medication within an appropriate time frame. Assess site, if possible, within 2 to 4 hours after administration.	

Skill Checklists to Accompany Fundamentals of Nursing:
The Art and Science of Nursing Care, 6th edition

Name _____ Date _____

Unit _____ Position _____

Instructor/Evaluator: _____ Position _____

SKILL 29-8
Adding Medications to an Intravenous (IV) Solution Container

Goal: The medication is added to an adequate amount of compatible solution and mixed appropriately.

Excellent	Satisfactory	Needs Practice		Comments
—	—	—	1. Gather equipment. Check medication order against the original physician's order according to agency policy. Clarify any inconsistencies. Check the patient's chart for allergies. Verify the compatibility of the medication and intravenous fluid. Calculate the infusion rate.	
—	—	—	2. Know the actions, special nursing considerations, safe dose ranges, purpose of administration, and adverse effects of the medications to be administered. Consider the appropriateness of the medication for this patient.	
—	—	—	3. Perform hand hygiene.	
—	—	—	4. Move the medication cart to the outside of the patient's room or prepare for administration in the medication area.	
—	—	—	5. Unlock the medication cart or drawer. Enter pass code and scan employee identification, if required.	
—	—	—	6. **Prepare medication for one patient at a time.**	
—	—	—	7. Read the MAR and select the proper medication from the patient's medication drawer or unit stock.	
—	—	—	8. Compare the label with the MAR. Check expiration dates and perform calculations, if necessary. Scan the barcode on the package, if required.	
—	—	—	9. If necessary, withdraw medication from an ampule or vial as described in Skills 29-2 and 29-3.	
—	—	—	10. **Recheck the label with the MAR before taking it to the patient.**	
—	—	—	11. Lock the medication cart before leaving it.	
—	—	—	12. Transport medications and equipment to the patient's bedside carefully, and keep the medications in sight at all times.	
—	—	—	13. Perform hand hygiene.	
—	—	—	14. **Identify the patient.** Usually, the patient should be identified using two methods. Compare information with the MAR or CMAR.	

Excellent	Satisfactory	Needs Practice		Comments
			SKILL 29-8 **Adding Medications to an Intravenous (IV)** **Solution Container** *(Continued)*	

Excellent	Satisfactory	Needs Practice		Comments
___	___	___	a. Check the name and identification number on the patient's identification band.	
___	___	___	b. Ask the patient to state his or her name.	
___	___	___	c. If the patient cannot identify him or herself, verify the patient's identification with a staff member who knows the patient for the second source.	
___	___	___	15. Close the door to the room or pull the bedside curtain.	
___	___	___	16. Complete necessary assessments before administering medications. Check allergy bracelet or ask patient about allergies. Explain the purpose and action of the medication to the patient.	
___	___	___	17. Scan the patient's barcode on the identification band, if required.	
___	___	___	18. **Check that the volume in the current intravenous infusion is adequate.**	
___	___	___	19. Close the clamp between the solution container and roller clamp on the infusion tubing and pause the intravenous pump, if appropriate.	
___	___	___	20. Clean the medication port with an antimicrobial swab.	
___	___	___	21. Steady the container and uncap the needle or needleless device. Insert it into the port. Inject the medication. Withdraw the needle or needleless device. Do not recap the used needle. Engage the safety shield or needle guard, if present.	
___	___	___	22. Remove the container from the IV pole and gently rotate the container to mix the medication and solution.	
___	___	___	23. Rehang the container on the pole. **Attach the label to the container so that the dose of medication that has been added is apparent.**	
___	___	___	24. Open the clamp, and readjust the flow rate or check the pump settings for correct infusion rate and restart pump.	
___	___	___	25. Discard the needle and syringe in the appropriate receptacle.	
___	___	___	26. Perform hand hygiene.	
___	___	___	27. Evaluate the patient's response to medication within the appropriate time frame.	

Skill Checklists to Accompany Fundamentals of Nursing:
The Art and Science of Nursing Care, 6th edition

Name _____   Date _____

Unit _____   Position _____

Instructor/Evaluator: _____   Position _____

Excellent	Satisfactory	Needs Practice	SKILL 29-9 **Administering Medications by Intravenous Bolus or Push Through an Intravenous Infusion**	
			Goal: The medication is given safely.	**Comments**
—	—	—	1. Gather equipment. Check medication order against the original physician's order according to agency policy. Clarify any inconsistencies. Check the patient's chart for allergies. Verify the compatibility of the medication and intravenous fluid. Check a drug resource to clarify whether medication needs to be diluted before administration. Check the infusion rate.	
—	—	—	2. Know the actions, special nursing considerations, safe dose ranges, purpose of administration, and adverse effects of the medications to be administered. Consider the appropriateness of the medication for this patient.	
—	—	—	3. Perform hand hygiene.	
—	—	—	4. Move the medication cart to the outside of the patient's room or prepare for administration in the medication area.	
—	—	—	5. Unlock the medication cart or drawer. Enter pass code and scan employee identification, if required.	
—	—	—	6. **Prepare medication for one patient at a time.**	
—	—	—	7. Read the MAR and select the proper medication from the patient's medication drawer or unit stock.	
—	—	—	8. Compare the label with the MAR. Check expiration dates and perform calculations, if necessary. Scan the barcode on the package, if required.	
—	—	—	9. If necessary, withdraw medication from an ampule or vial as described in Skills 29-2 and 29-3.	
—	—	—	10. **Recheck the label with the MAR before taking it to the patient.**	
—	—	—	11. Lock the medication cart before leaving it.	
—	—	—	12. Transport medications and equipment to the patient's bedside carefully, and keep the medications in sight at all times.	
—	—	—	13. Perform hand hygiene.	
—	—	—	14. **Identify the patient.** Usually, the patient should be identified using two methods. Compare information with the MAR or CMAR.	

SKILL 29-9

Administering Medications by Intravenous Bolus or Push Through an Intravenous Infusion *(Continued)*

Excellent	Satisfactory	Needs Practice		Comments
___	___	___	a. Check the name and identification number on the patient's identification band.	
___	___	___	b. Ask the patient to state his or her name.	
___	___	___	c. If the patient cannot identify him or herself, verify the patient's identification with a staff member who knows the patient for the second source.	
___	___	___	15. Close the door to the room or pull the bedside curtain.	
___	___	___	16. Complete necessary assessments before administering medications. Check allergy bracelet or ask patient about allergies. Explain the purpose and action of the medication to the patient.	
___	___	___	17. Scan the patient's barcode on the identification band, if required.	
___	___	___	18. **Assess IV site for presence of inflammation or infiltration.**	
___	___	___	19. If IV infusion is being administered via an infusion pump, pause the pump.	
___	___	___	20. Put on clean gloves.	
___	___	___	21. Select injection port on tubing that is closest to venipuncture site. Clean port with antimicrobial swab.	
___	___	___	22. Uncap syringe. Steady port with your nondominant hand while inserting syringe, needleless device, or needle into center of port.	
___	___	___	23. Move your nondominant hand to the section of IV tubing just above the injection port. Fold tubing between your fingers.	
___	___	___	24. Pull back slightly on plunger just until blood appears in tubing.	
___	___	___	25. **Inject medication at recommended rate.**	
___	___	___	26. Release the tubing. Remove the syringe. Do not recap the used needle. Engage the safety shield or needle guard, if present. Release the tubing and allow the IV fluid to flow. Discard the needle and syringe in the appropriate receptacle.	
___	___	___	27. Check IV fluid infusion rate. Restart infusion pump, if appropriate.	
___	___	___	28. Remove gloves and perform hand hygiene.	
___	___	___	29. Evaluate patient's response to medication within appropriate time frame.	

Skill Checklists to Accompany Fundamentals of Nursing:
The Art and Science of Nursing Care, 6th edition

Name _____   Date _____

Unit _____   Position _____

Instructor/Evaluator: _____   Position _____

SKILL 29-10

Administering Intravenous Medications by Piggyback, Mini-Infusion Pump, or Volume Control Administration Set

Goal: The medication is delivered via the parenteral route using sterile technique.

Excellent	Satisfactory	Needs Practice		Comments
___	___	___	1. Gather equipment. Check each medication order against the original physician's order according to agency policy. Clarify any inconsistencies. Check the patient's chart for allergies.	
___	___	___	2. Know the actions, special nursing considerations, safe dose ranges, purpose of administration, and adverse effects of the medications to be administered. Consider the appropriateness of the medication for this patient.	
___	___	___	3. Perform hand hygiene.	
___	___	___	4. Move the medication cart to the outside of the patient's room or prepare for administration in the medication area.	
___	___	___	5. Unlock the medication cart or drawer. Enter pass code and scan employee identification, if required.	
___	___	___	6. **Prepare medications for one patient at a time.**	
___	___	___	7. Read the MAR and select the proper medication from the patient's medication drawer or unit stock.	
___	___	___	8. Compare the label with the MAR. Check expiration dates. Confirm the prescribed or appropriate infusion rate. Calculate the drip rate if using gravity system. Scan the barcode on the package, if required.	
___	___	___	9. **When all medications for one patient have been prepared, recheck the label with the MAR before taking them to the patient.**	
___	___	___	10. Lock the medication cart before leaving it.	
___	___	___	11. Transport medications to the patient's bedside carefully, and keep the medications in sight at all times.	
___	___	___	12. **Ensure that the patient receives the medications at the correct time.**	
___	___	___	13. **Identify the patient.** Usually, the patient should be identified using two methods. Compare information with the MAR or CMAR.	

Excellent	Satisfactory	Needs Practice	SKILL 29-10 **Administering Intravenous Medications by Piggyback, Mini-Infusion Pump, or Volume Control Administration Set** *(Continued)*	Comments
——	——	——	a. Check the name and identification number on the patient's identification band.	
——	——	——	b. Ask the patient to state his or her name.	
——	——	——	c. If the patient cannot identify him or herself, verify the patient's identification with a staff member who knows the patient for the second source.	
——	——	——	14. Close the door to the room or pull the bedside curtain.	
——	——	——	15. Perform hand hygiene.	
——	——	——	16. Complete necessary assessments before administering medications. Check allergy bracelet or ask patient about allergies. Explain the purpose and action of the medication to the patient.	
——	——	——	17. Scan the patient's barcode on the identification band, if required.	
——	——	——	18. Assess the IV site for the presence of inflammation or infiltration.	
			For a Piggyback Infusion	
——	——	——	19. Close the clamp on the short secondary infusion tubing. Using aseptic technique, remove the cap on the tubing spike and the cap on the port of the medication container, taking care to not contaminate either end.	
——	——	——	20. Attach infusion tubing to the medication container by inserting the tubing spike into the port with a firm push and twisting motion, taking care to not contaminate either end.	
——	——	——	21. **Hang piggyback container on IV pole, positioning it higher than primary IV according to manufacturer's recommendations.** Use metal or plastic hook to lower primary intravenous fluid container.	
——	——	——	22. Place label on tubing with appropriate date.	
——	——	——	23. Squeeze drip chamber and release. Fill to the line or about half full. Open clamp and prime tubing. Close clamp. Place needleless connector or needle on the end of the tubing, using sterile technique, if required.	
——	——	——	24. Use an antimicrobial swab to clean the access port or stopcock above the roller clamp on the primary IV infusion tubing.	
——	——	——	25. Connect piggyback setup to the access port or stopcock. If using, turn the stopcock to the open position.	

SKILL 29-10
Administering Intravenous Medications by Piggyback, Mini-Infusion Pump, or Volume Control Administration Set *(Continued)*

Excellent	Satisfactory	Needs Practice		Comments

Comments

Excellent	Satisfactory	Needs Practice	
——	——	——	26. Use strip of tape to secure secondary tubing to primary infusion tubing, if a needle is used to connect.
——	——	——	27. Open clamp on the secondary tubing. Use the roller clamp on the primary infusion tubing to regulate flow at the prescribed delivery rate or set rate for secondary infusion on infusion pump. Monitor medication infusion at periodic intervals.
——	——	——	28. Clamp tubing on piggyback set when solution is infused. Follow agency policy regarding disposal of equipment.
——	——	——	29. Replace primary IV fluid container to original height. **Readjust flow rate of primary IV or check primary infusion rate on infusion pump.** Proceed to step 51.

For a Mini-Infusion Pump

——	——	——	30. Using aseptic technique, remove the cap on the tubing and the cap on the syringe, taking care to not contaminate either end.
——	——	——	31. Attach infusion tubing to the syringe, taking care to not contaminate either end.
——	——	——	32. Place label on tubing with appropriate date and attach needle or needleless device to end of tubing according to manufacturer's directions.
——	——	——	33. Fill tubing with medication by applying gentle pressure to syringe plunger. Place needleless connector or needle on the end of the tubing, using sterile technique, if required.
——	——	——	34. Insert syringe into mini-infusion pump according to manufacturer's directions.
——	——	——	35. Use antimicrobial swab to clean the access port or stopcock below the roller clamp on the primary IV infusion tubing, usually the port closest to the IV insertion site.
——	——	——	36. Connect the secondary infusion to the primary infusion at the cleansed port.
——	——	——	37. Program pump to the appropriate rate and begin infusion. Set alarm if recommended by manufacturer.
——	——	——	38. Clamp tubing on secondary set when solution is infused. Remove secondary tubing from access port and replace connector or needle with a new, capped one, if reusing. Follow agency policy regarding disposal of equipment.
——	——	——	39. Check rate of primary infusion. Proceed to step 51.

SKILL 29-10

Administering Intravenous Medications by Piggyback, Mini-Infusion Pump, or Volume Control Administration Set *(Continued)*

Excellent	Satisfactory	Needs Practice		Comments

For a Volume-Control Administration Set

40. Fill the volume-control administration set with the prescribed amount of intravenous fluid by opening the clamp between IV solution and the volume-control administration set. Follow manufacturer's instructions and fill with prescribed amount of IV solution. Close clamp.

41. Check to make sure the air vent on the volume-control administration set chamber is open.

42. Use antimicrobial swab to clean access port on volume-control administration set chamber.

43. Insert the needle or blunt needleless device into the port while holding syringe steady. Inject medication into the chamber. Gently rotate the chamber.

44. Attach the medication label to the volume-control device.

45. Use antimicrobial swab to clean the access port or stopcock below the roller clamp on the primary IV infusion tubing, usually the port closest to the IV insertion site.

46. Connect the secondary infusion to the primary infusion at the cleansed port.

47. Use the roller clamp on the volume-control administration set tubing to adjust the infusion to the prescribed rate.

48. Do not recap the used needle. Engage the safety shield or needle guard, if present. Discard the needle and syringe in the appropriate receptacle.

49. Clamp tubing on secondary set when solution is infused. Remove secondary tubing from access port and replace connector or needle with a new, capped one, if reusing. Follow agency policy regarding disposal of equipment.

50. Check rate of primary infusion.

51. Perform hand hygiene.

52. Evaluate patient's response to medication within appropriate time frame. Monitor IV site at periodic intervals.

Skill Checklists to Accompany Fundamentals of Nursing:
The Art and Science of Nursing Care, 6th edition

Name _____ Date _____

Unit _____ Position _____

Instructor/Evaluator: _____ Position _____

SKILL 29-11

Introducing Drugs Through a Medication or Drug Infusion Lock Using the Saline Flush (Intermittent Peripheral Venous Access Device)

Goal: The medication is delivered via the parenteral route using sterile technique.

Excellent	Satisfactory	Needs Practice		Comments
——	——	——	1. Gather equipment. Check medication order against the original physician's order according to agency policy. Clarify any inconsistencies. Check the patient's chart for allergies. Verify the compatibility of the medication and intravenous fluid. Check a drug resource to clarify whether medication needs to be diluted before administration. Check the infusion rate.	
——	——	——	2. Know the actions, special nursing considerations, safe dose ranges, purpose of administration, and adverse effects of the medications to be administered. Consider the appropriateness of the medication for this patient.	
——	——	——	3. Perform hand hygiene.	
——	——	——	4. Move the medication cart to the outside of the patient's room or prepare for administration in the medication area.	
——	——	——	5. Unlock the medication cart or drawer. Enter pass code and scan employee identification, if required.	
——	——	——	6. **Prepare medication for one patient at a time.**	
——	——	——	7. Read the MAR and select the proper medication from the patient's medication drawer or unit stock.	
——	——	——	8. Compare the label with the MAR. Check expiration dates and perform calculations, if necessary. Scan the barcode on the package, if required.	
——	——	——	9. If necessary, withdraw medication from an ampule or vial as described in Skills 29-2 and 29-3.	
——	——	——	10. **Recheck the label with the MAR before taking it to the patient.**	
——	——	——	11. Lock the medication cart before leaving it.	
——	——	——	12. Transport medications and equipment to the patient's bedside carefully, and keep the medications in sight at all times.	
——	——	——	13. Perform hand hygiene.	

SKILL 29-11

Introducing Drugs Through a Medication or Drug Infusion Lock Using the Saline Flush (Intermittent Peripheral Venous Access Device) *(Continued)*

Excellent	Satisfactory	Needs Practice		Comments
——	——	——	14. **Identify the patient.** Usually, the patient should be identified using two methods. Compare information with the MAR or CMAR.	
——	——	——	a. Check the name and identification number on the patient's identification band.	
——	——	——	b. Ask the patient to state his or her name.	
——	——	——	c. If the patient cannot identify him or herself, verify the patient's identification with a staff member who knows the patient for the second source.	
——	——	——	15. Close the door to the room or pull the bedside curtain.	
——	——	——	16. Complete necessary assessments before administering medications. Check allergy bracelet or ask patient about allergies. Explain the purpose and action of the medication to the patient.	
——	——	——	17. Scan the patient's barcode on the identification band, if required.	
——	——	——	18. **Assess IV site for presence of inflammation or infiltration.**	
——	——	——	19. Put on clean gloves.	
——	——	——	20. Clean the access port of the medication lock with antimicrobial swab.	
——	——	——	21. Stabilize port with your nondominant hand and insert needleless device, syringe, or needle of syringe of normal saline into access port.	
——	——	——	22. Release the clamp on the extension tubing of the medication lock. Aspirate gently and check for blood return.	
——	——	——	23. Gently flush with normal saline by pushing slowly on the syringe plunger. Observe the insertion site while inserting the saline. Remove syringe.	
——	——	——	24. Insert needleless device or needle of syringe with medication into port and gently inject medication, using a watch to verify correct administration rate. **Do not force the injection if resistance is felt.**	
——	——	——	25. Remove medication syringe from port. Stabilize port with your nondominant hand and insert needleless device or needle of syringe of normal saline into port. Gently flush with normal saline by pushing slowly on the syringe plunger. To gain positive pressure, clamp the IV tubing as you are still flushing the last of the saline into the medication lock. Remove syringe.	

46

Excellent	Satisfactory	Needs Practice		Comments

SKILL 29-11

Introducing Drugs Through a Medication or Drug Infusion Lock Using the Saline Flush (Intermittent Peripheral Venous Access Device) *(Continued)*

Excellent	Satisfactory	Needs Practice		Comments
——	——	——	26. Do not recap the used needle. Engage the safety shield or needle guard, if present. Discard the needle and syringe in the appropriate receptacle.	
——	——	——	27. Remove gloves and perform hand hygiene.	
——	——	——	28. Evaluate patient's response to medication within appropriate time frame.	
——	——	——	29. Check medication lock site at least every 8 hours or according to facility policy.	

Skill Checklists to Accompany Fundamentals of Nursing:
The Art and Science of Nursing Care, 6th edition

Name _____   Date _____

Unit _____   Position _____

Instructor/Evaluator: _____   Position _____

Excellent	Satisfactory	Needs Practice	SKILL 29-12 **Administering an Eye Irrigation**	
			Goal: The eye is cleansed successfully.	**Comments**
——	——	——	1. Gather equipment. Check the original physician's order for the irrigation according to agency policy. Clarify any inconsistencies. Check the patient's chart for allergies.	
——	——	——	2. **Identify the patient.** Usually, the patient should be identified using two methods. Compare information with the MAR or CMAR.	
——	——	——	a. Check the name and identification number on the patient's identification band.	
——	——	——	b. Ask the patient to state his or her name.	
——	——	——	c. If the patient cannot identify him or herself, verify the patient's identification with a staff member who knows the patient for the second source.	
——	——	——	3. Explain the procedure to patient.	
——	——	——	4. Assemble equipment at the patient's bedside.	
——	——	——	5. Perform hand hygiene.	
——	——	——	6. Have patient sit or lie with head tilted toward side of affected eye. Protect patient and bed with a waterproof pad.	
——	——	——	7. Put on disposable gloves. Clean lids and lashes with washcloth moistened with normal saline or the solution ordered for the irrigation. Wipe from inner canthus to outer canthus. Use a different corner of washcloth with each wipe.	
——	——	——	8. Place curved basin at cheek on side of affected eye to receive irrigating solution. If patient is able, ask him or her to support the basin.	
——	——	——	9. Expose lower conjunctival sac and hold upper lid open with your nondominant hand.	
——	——	——	10. Fill the irrigation syringe with the prescribed fluid. **Hold irrigation syringe about 2.5 cm (1″) from eye. Direct flow of solution from inner to outer canthus along conjunctival sac.**	

Excellent	Satisfactory	Needs Practice	SKILL 29-12 **Administering an Eye Irrigation** *(Continued)*	Comments
——	——	——	11. Irrigate until the solution is clear or all the solution has been used. **Use only enough force to remove secretions gently from the conjunctiva. Avoid touching any part of the eye with the irrigating tip.**	
——	——	——	12. Pause irrigation and have patient close eye periodically during procedure.	
——	——	——	13. Dry periorbital area after irrigation with gauze sponge. Offer towel to patient if face and neck are wet.	
——	——	——	14. Remove gloves and perform hand hygiene.	
——	——	——	15. Assist the patient to a comfortable position.	
——	——	——	16. Evaluate patient's response to medication within appropriate time frame.	

Skill Checklists to Accompany Fundamentals of Nursing:
The Art and Science of Nursing Care, 6th edition

Name _____   Date _____

Unit _____   Position _____

Instructor/Evaluator: _____   Position _____

Excellent	Satisfactory	Needs Practice	SKILL 29-13 **Administering an Ear Irrigation**	Comments
			Goal: The irrigation is administered successfully.	
____	____	____	1. Gather equipment. Check the original physician's order for the irrigation according to agency policy. Clarify any inconsistencies. Check the patient's chart for allergies.	
____	____	____	2. **Identify the patient.** Usually, the patient should be identified using two methods. Compare information with the MAR or CMAR.	
____	____	____	a. Check the name and identification number on the patient's identification band.	
____	____	____	b. Ask the patient to state his or her name.	
____	____	____	c. If the patient cannot identify him or herself, verify the patient's identification with a staff member who knows the patient for the second source.	
____	____	____	3. Explain procedure to patient.	
____	____	____	4. Assemble equipment at the patient's bedside.	
____	____	____	5. Perform hand hygiene and put on gloves.	
____	____	____	6. Have patient sit up or lie with head tilted toward side of affected ear. Protect patient and bed with a waterproof pad. Have patient support basin under the ear to receive the irrigating solution.	
____	____	____	7. Clean pinna and meatus of auditory canal as necessary with moistened cotton-tipped applicators dipped in warm tap water or the irrigating solution.	
____	____	____	8. Fill bulb syringe with warm solution. If an irrigating container is used, prime the tubing.	
____	____	____	9. Straighten auditory canal by pulling cartilaginous portion of pinna up and back for an adult.	
____	____	____	10. **Direct a steady, slow stream of solution against the roof of the auditory canal, using only enough force to remove secretions. Do not occlude the auditory canal with the irrigating nozzle. Allow solution to flow out unimpeded.**	
____	____	____	11. When irrigation is complete, place cotton ball loosely in auditory meatus and have the patient lie on side of affected ear on a towel or absorbent pad.	

SKILL 29-13
Administering an Ear Irrigation *(Continued)*

Excellent	Satisfactory	Needs Practice		Comments
——	——	——	12. Remove gloves and perform hand hygiene.	
——	——	——	13. Assist the patient to a comfortable position.	
——	——	——	14. Evaluate the patient's response to the procedure. Return in 10 to 15 minutes and remove cotton ball and assess drainage.	

Skill Checklists to Accompany Fundamentals of Nursing:
The Art and Science of Nursing Care, 6th edition

Name _____   Date _____

Unit _____   Position _____

Instructor/Evaluator: _____   Position _____

SKILL 30-1
Providing Preoperative Patient Care: Hospitalized Patient

Goal: The patient will proceed to surgery, be free from anxiety and fear, and demonstrate an understanding of the need for surgery and measures to minimize the postoperative risks associated with surgery.

Excellent	Satisfactory	Needs Practice		Comments
___	___	___	1. Check the patient's chart for the type of surgery and review the physician's orders. Review the nursing database, history, and physical examination. Check that the baseline data are recorded; report those that are abnormal.	
___	___	___	2. **Check that diagnostic testing has been completed and results are available; identify and report abnormal results.**	
___	___	___	3. Gather needed equipment and supplies.	
___	___	___	4. Perform hand hygiene.	
___	___	___	5. Identify the patient.	
___	___	___	6. Explore the psychological needs of the patient related to the surgery as well as the family.	
___	___	___	a. Establish the therapeutic relationship encouraging the patient to verbalize concerns or fears.	
___	___	___	b. Use active learning skills, answering questions and clarifying any misinformation.	
___	___	___	c. Use touch, as appropriate, to convey genuine empathy.	
___	___	___	d. Offer to contact spiritual counselor (priest, minister, rabbi) to meet spiritual needs.	
___	___	___	7. **Identify learning needs of patient and family.** Ensure that the informed consent of the patient for the surgery has been signed, witnessed and dated. Inquire if the patient has any questions regarding the surgical procedure. Check the patient's record to determine if an advance directive has been completed. If an advance directive has not been completed, discuss with the patient the possibility of completing as appropriate. If patient has had surgery before, ask about this experience.	
___	___	___	8. Provide teaching about deep-breathing exercises.	
___	___	___	9. Conduct teaching regarding coughing and splinting (providing support to the incision).	
___	___	___	10. Provide teaching regarding incentive spirometer.	

Excellent	Satisfactory	Needs Practice		Comments

11. Provide teaching regarding leg exercises.

    a. Assist or ask the patient to sit up (semi-Fowler's position) and explain to patient that you will first demonstrate, and then coach him/her to exercise one leg at a time.

    b. Straighten the patient's knee, raise the foot, extend the lower leg, and hold this position for a few seconds. Lower the entire leg. Practice this exercise with the other leg.

    c. Assist or ask the patient to point the toes of both legs toward the foot of the bed then relax them. Next, flex or pull the toes toward the chin.

    d. Assist or ask the patient to keep legs extended and to make circles with both ankles, first circling to the left and then to the right. Instruct the patient to repeat these exercises 3 times.

12. Assist the patient in putting on antiembolism stockings and demonstrate how the pneumatic compression device operates.

13. Provide teaching regarding turning in the bed.

    a. Instruct the patient to use a pillow or bath blanket to splint where the incision will be. Ask the patient to raise his or her left knee and reach across to grasp the right side rail of the bed when he/she is turning toward his or her right side. If patient is turning to his or her left side, he or she will bend the right knee and grasp the left side rail.

    b. When turning the patient onto his or her right side, ask the patient to push with bent left leg and pull on the right side rail. Explain to the patient that the nurse will place a pillow behind his/her back to provide support and that the call bell will be placed within easy reach.

    c. Explain to the patient that position change is recommended every 2 hours.

14. Provide teaching about pain management.

    a. Discuss past experiences with pain and interventions that the patient has used to reduce pain.

    b. Discuss the availability of analgesic medication postoperatively.

Excellent	Satisfactory	Needs Practice	SKILL 30-1 **Providing Preoperative Patient Care:** **Hospitalized Patient** *(Continued)*	Comments
___	___	___	c. Explore the use of other alternative and nonpharmacological methods to reduce pain, such as position change, massage, relaxation/diversion, guided imagery, and meditation.	
___	___	___	15. Review equipment.	
___	___	___	a. Show the patient the various equipment such as IV pumps, electronic blood pressure cuff, tubes, and surgical drains.	
___	___	___	16. Provide skin preparation.	
___	___	___	a. **Ask the patient to shower with the antiseptic solution. Remind the patient to carefully clean around the surgical site.**	
___	___	___	b. **For site-specific surgery, such as a leg, ask the patient to mark the correct site with a marker.**	
___	___	___	17. Provide teaching about and follow dietary/fluid restrictions.	
___	___	___	a. **Explain to the patient that both food and fluid will be restricted prior to surgery to ensure that the stomach contains a minimal amount of gastric secretions. This restriction is important to reduce the risk of aspiration. Emphasize to the patient the importance of avoiding food and fluids during the prescribed time period since failure to adhere may necessitate cancellation of the surgery.**	
___	___	___	18. Provide intestinal preparation. In certain situations, the bowel will need to be prepared through the administering of enemas or laxatives to evacuate the bowel and to reduce the intestinal bacteria.	
___	___	___	a. **As needed, provide explanation of the purpose of enemas or laxatives prior to surgery. If the patient will be administering an enema, clarify the steps as needed.**	
___	___	___	19. **Check administration of regularly scheduled medications.** Review with patient routine medications, over-the-counter, and other herbal supplements that are taken regularly. Check the physician's orders and review with the patient which medications he/she will be permitted to take the day of surgery.	
___	___	___	20. Perform hand hygiene.	

Skill Checklists to Accompany Fundamentals of Nursing:
The Art and Science of Nursing Care, 6th edition

Name _____ Date _____

Unit _____ Position _____

Instructor/Evaluator: _____ Position _____

Excellent	Satisfactory	Needs Practice	SKILL 30-2 **Providing Postoperative Care When Patient Returns to Room**	Comments
			Goal: The patient will recover from the surgery, free of complications.	
			Immediate Care	
____	____	____	1. When patient returns from the PACU, obtain a report from the PACU nurse and review the operating room and PACU data.	
____	____	____	2. Perform hand hygiene.	
____	____	____	3. Identify the patient.	
____	____	____	4. **Place patient in safe position (semi- or high Fowler's or side-lying). Note level of consciousness.**	
____	____	____	5. **Obtain vital signs. Monitor and record vital signs frequently.** Assessment order may vary, but usual frequency includes taking vital signs every 15 minutes the first hour, every 30 minutes the next 2 hours, every hour for 4 hours, and finally every 4 hours.	
____	____	____	6. Provide for warmth, using heated blankets as necessary. Assess skin color and condition.	
____	____	____	7. **Check dressings for color, odor, presence of drains, and amount of drainage. Mark the drainage on the dressing by circulating the amount and include the time. Assess under the patient for bleeding from the surgical site.**	
____	____	____	8. **Verify that all tubes and drains are patent and equipment is operative; note amount of drainage in collection device. If Foley catheter is in place, note urinary output.**	
____	____	____	9. Maintain IV infusion at the correct rate.	
____	____	____	10. Provide for a safe environment. Keep bed in low position with side rails up. Have call bell within patient's reach.	
____	____	____	11. Assess for and relieve pain by administering medications ordered by the physician. If the patient has been instructed in the use of PCA for pain management, review use. Check record to verify if analgesic medication was administered in the PACU.	
____	____	____	12. Record assessments and interventions on chart.	

Excellent	Satisfactory	Needs Practice		
			SKILL 30-2 **Providing Postoperative Care When Patient Returns to Room** *(Continued)*	
				Comments
			Ongoing Care	
——	——	——	13. Promote optimal respiratory function.	
——	——	——	a. Assess respiratory rate, depth, quality, color, and capillary refill. Ask if patient is experiencing any difficulty breathing.	
——	——	——	b. Assist with coughing and deep-breathing exercises.	
——	——	——	c. Assist with incentive spirometry.	
——	——	——	d. Assist with early ambulation.	
——	——	——	e. Provide frequent position change.	
——	——	——	f. Administer oxygen as ordered.	
——	——	——	g. Monitor pulse oximetry.	
——	——	——	14. Promote optimal cardiovascular function:	
——	——	——	a. Assess apical rate, rhythm, and quality and compare to peripheral pulses, color, and blood pressure. Ask if the patient has any chest pains or shortness of breath.	
——	——	——	b. Provide frequent position changes.	
——	——	——	c. Assist with early ambulation.	
——	——	——	d. Apply antiembolism stockings or pneumatic compression devices, if ordered by physician.	
——	——	——	e. Provide leg and range-of-motion exercises if not contraindicated.	
——	——	——	15. Promote optimal neurological function:	
——	——	——	a. Assess level of consciousness, motor function, and sensation.	
——	——	——	b. Determine the level of orientation to person, place, and time.	
——	——	——	c. Test motor ability by asking the patient to move each extremity	
——	——	——	d. Evaluate sensation by asking the patient if he/she can feel your touch on an extremity.	
——	——	——	16. **Promote optimal renal and urinary function and fluid and electrolyte status. Assess intake and output, for urinary retention and serum electrolytes.**	
——	——	——	a. Promote voiding by offering bedpan at regular intervals noting the frequency, amount, and if any burning or urgency symptoms.	

56

Excellent	Satisfactory	Needs Practice		Comments

SKILL 30-2
Providing Postoperative Care When Patient Returns to Room *(Continued)*

—— —— ——		b. Monitor urinary catheter drainage if present.	
—— —— ——		c. Measure intake and output.	
—— —— ——		17. Promote optimal gastrointestinal function and meet nutritional needs:	
—— —— ——		a. Assess abdomen for distention, firmness. Ask if patient feels nauseated, has any vomiting, or is passing flatus.	
—— —— ——		b. Auscultate for bowel sounds.	
—— —— ——		c. Assist with diet progression.	
—— —— ——		d. Encourage fluid intake.	
—— —— ——		e. Monitor intake.	
—— —— ——		f. Medicate for nausea and vomiting as ordered by physician.	
—— —— ——		18. Promote optimal wound healing.	
—— —— ——		a. Assess condition of wound, for presence of drains and any drainage.	
—— —— ——		b. Use surgical asepsis for dressing changes.	
—— —— ——		c. Inspect all skin surfaces for beginning signs of pressure ulcer development and utilize pressure-relieving supports to minimize potential skin breakdown.	
—— —— ——		19. Promote optimal comfort and relief from pain.	
—— —— ——		a. Assess for pain (location, intensity using scale).	
—— —— ——		b. Provide for rest and comfort.	
—— —— ——		c. Administer pain medications as needed or other nonpharmacologic methods.	
—— —— ——		20. Promote optimal meeting of psychosocial needs:	
—— —— ——		a. Provide emotional support to patient and family as needed.	
—— —— ——		b. Explain procedures and offer explanations regarding postoperative recovery, as needed, to both patient and family members.	

Skill Checklists to Accompany Fundamentals of Nursing:
The Art and Science of Nursing Care, 6th edition

Name _____   Date _____

Unit _____   Position _____

Instructor/Evaluator: _____   Position _____

Excellent	Satisfactory	Needs Practice	SKILL 37-1 **Giving a Bed Bath**	
			Goal: The patient will be clean and fresh.	**Comments**
——	——	——	1. Review chart for any limitations in physical activity. Identify the patient. Discuss procedure with the patient and assess the patient's ability to assist in the bathing process, as well as personal hygiene preferences.	
——	——	——	2. Bring necessary equipment to the bedside stand or overbed table. Remove sequential compression devices and antiembolism stockings from lower extremities according to agency protocol.	
——	——	——	3. Close curtains around bed and close door to room if possible. Adjust the room temperature if necessary.	
——	——	——	4. Offer the patient a bedpan or urinal.	
——	——	——	5. Perform hand hygiene.	
——	——	——	6. Raise bed to a comfortable working height.	
——	——	——	7. Lower side rail nearer to you and assist the patient to the side of bed where you will work. Have the patient lie on his or her back.	
——	——	——	8. Loosen top covers and remove all except the top sheet. Place bath blanket over the patient and then remove top sheet while the patient holds bath blanket in place. If linen is to be reused, fold it over a chair. Place soiled linen in laundry bag. Take care to prevent linen from coming in contact with your clothing.	
——	——	——	9. Remove the patient's gown and keep bath blanket in place. If the patient has an IV line and is not wearing a gown with snap sleeves, remove gown from other arm first. **Lower the IV container and pass gown over the tubing and the container. Rehang the container and check the drip rate.**	
——	——	——	10. **Raise side rail.** Fill basin with a sufficient amount of comfortably warm water (110°–115°F). Change as necessary throughout the bath. Lower side rail closer to you when you return to the bedside to begin the bath.	

Excellent	Satisfactory	Needs Practice	SKILL 37-1 **Giving a Bed Bath** *(Continued)*
			Comments
⎯	⎯	⎯	11. Put on gloves, if necessary. Fold the washcloth like a mitt on your hand so that there are no loose ends.
⎯	⎯	⎯	12. Lay a towel across the patient's chest and on top of bath blanket.
⎯	⎯	⎯	13. **With no soap on the washcloth, wipe one eye from the inner part of the eye, near the nose, to the outer part. Rinse or turn the cloth before washing the other eye.**
⎯	⎯	⎯	14. Bathe the patient's face, neck, and ears, avoiding soap on the face if the patient prefers. Apply appropriate emollient.
⎯	⎯	⎯	15. Expose the patient's far arm and place towel lengthwise under it. Using firm strokes, wash arm and axilla, lifting the arm as necessary to access axillary region. Rinse, if necessary, and dry. Apply appropriate emollient.
⎯	⎯	⎯	16. Place a folded towel on the bed next to the patient's hand and put basin on it. Soak the patient's hand in basin. Wash, rinse, if necessary, and dry hand. Apply appropriate emollient.
⎯	⎯	⎯	17. Repeat Actions 15 and 16 for the arm nearer you. An option for the shorter nurse or one prone to back strain might be to bathe one side of the patient and move to the other side of the bed to complete the bath.
⎯	⎯	⎯	18. Spread a towel across the patient's chest. Lower bath blanket to the patient's umbilical area. Wash, rinse, if necessary, and dry chest. Keep chest covered with towel between the wash and rinse. Pay special attention to skin folds under the breasts.
⎯	⎯	⎯	19. Lower bath blanket to perineal area. Place a towel over the patient's chest.
⎯	⎯	⎯	20. Wash, rinse, if necessary, and dry abdomen. Carefully inspect and cleanse umbilical area and any abdominal folds or creases.
⎯	⎯	⎯	21. Return bath blanket to original position and expose far leg. Place towel under far leg. Using firm strokes, wash, rinse, if necessary, and dry leg from ankle to knee and knee to groin. Apply appropriate emollient.
⎯	⎯	⎯	22. Fold a towel near the patient's foot area and place basin on it. Place foot in basin while supporting the ankle and heel in your hand and the leg on your arm. Wash, rinse, if necessary, and dry, paying particular attention to area between toes. Apply appropriate emollient.

Giving a Bed Bath *(Continued)*

Excellent	Satisfactory	Needs Practice		Comments
——	——	——	23. Repeat Actions 21 and 22 for the other leg and foot.	
——	——	——	24. Make sure the patient is covered with the bath blanket. Change water and washcloth at this point or earlier if necessary.	
——	——	——	25. Assist the patient to prone or side-lying position. Put on gloves, if not applied earlier. Position bath blanket and towel to expose only the back and buttocks.	
——	——	——	26. Wash, rinse, if necessary, and dry the back and buttocks area. **Pay particular attention to cleansing between gluteal folds, and observe for any redness or skin breakdown in the sacral area.**	
——	——	——	27. If not contraindicated, give the patient a backrub, as described in Chapter 10. Back massage may be given also after perineal care. Apply an appropriate emollient and/or skin barrier product.	
——	——	——	28. Raise the side rail. Refill basin with clean water. Discard washcloth and towel. Remove gloves and put on clean gloves.	
——	——	——	29. Clean perineal area or set up the patient so that he or she can complete perineal self-care. If the patient is unable, lower the side rail and complete perineal care, following guidelines given in the chapter text. Raise side rail, remove gloves, and perform hand hygiene.	
——	——	——	30. Help the patient put on a clean gown and assist with the use of other personal toiletries, such as deodorant or cosmetics.	
——	——	——	31. Protect the pillow with a towel and groom the patient's hair.	
——	——	——	32. Change bed linens, as described in Skills 37-5 and 37-6. Remove gloves and perform hand hygiene. Dispose of soiled linens according to agency policy.	

Skill Checklists to Accompany Fundamentals of Nursing:
The Art and Science of Nursing Care, 6th edition

Name _____   Date _____

Unit _____   Position _____

Instructor/Evaluator: _____   Position _____

SKILL 37-2

Assisting the Patient With Oral Care

Goal: The patient's mouth and teeth will be clean; the patient will exhibit a positive body image; and the patient will verbalize the importance of oral care.

Excellent	Satisfactory	Needs Practice		Comments
——	——	——	1. Identify the patient. Explain procedure to the patient.	
——	——	——	2. Perform hand hygiene. Put on disposable gloves if assisting with oral care.	
——	——	——	3. Assemble equipment on an overbed table within the patient's reach.	
——	——	——	4. Provide privacy for the patient.	
——	——	——	5. Lower side rail and assist the patient to sitting position if permitted, or turn the patient onto side. Place towel across the patient's chest. Raise bed to a comfortable working position.	
——	——	——	6. Encourage the patient to brush his/her own teeth, or assist if necessary.	
——	——	——	a. Moisten the toothbrush and apply toothpaste to bristles.	
——	——	——	b. Place the brush at a 45-degree angle to the gum line and brush from the gum line to the crown of each too. Brush outer and inner surfaces. Brush back and forth across the biting surface of each tooth.	
——	——	——	c. Brush the tongue gently with the toothbrush.	
——	——	——	d. Have the patient rinse vigorously with water and spit into the emesis basin. Repeat until clear. Suction may be used as an alternative for removal of fluid and secretions from mouth.	
——	——	——	7. Assist the patient to floss teeth, if appropriate:	
——	——	——	a. Remove approximately 6″ of dental floss from container or use a plastic floss holder. Wrap the floss around the index fingers, keeping about 1″ to 1.5″ of floss taut between the fingers.	
——	——	——	b. Insert floss gently between teeth, moving it back and forth downward to the gums.	
——	——	——	c. Move the floss up and down first on one side of a tooth and then on the side of the other tooth, until the surfaces are clean. Repeat in the spaces between all teeth.	

Assisting the Patient With Oral Care *(Continued)*

Excellent	Satisfactory	Needs Practice		Comments
——	——	——	d. Instruct patient to rinse mouth well with water after flossing.	
——	——	——	8. Offer mouthwash if patient prefers.	
——	——	——	9. Offer lip balm or petroleum jelly.	
——	——	——	10. Remove equipment. Remove gloves and discard. Raise side rail and lower bed. Assist the patient to a position of comfort.	
——	——	——	11. Perform hand hygiene.	

Skill Checklists to Accompany Fundamentals of Nursing:
The Art and Science of Nursing Care, 6th edition

Name _____   Date _____

Unit _____   Position _____

Instructor/Evaluator: _____   Position _____

Excellent	Satisfactory	Needs Practice	SKILL 37-3 **Providing Oral Care for the Dependent Patient**	
			Goal: The patient's mouth and teeth will be clean.	**Comments**
——	——	——	1. Identify the patient. Explain the procedure to the patient.	
——	——	——	2. Perform hand hygiene and put on disposable gloves.	
——	——	——	3. Assemble equipment on an overbed table within reach.	
——	——	——	4. Provide privacy for the patient. Adjust height of bed to a comfortable position. Lower one side rail and position the patient on the side, with head tilted forward. Place towel across the patient's chest and emesis basin in position under the chin.	
——	——	——	5. Open the patient's mouth and gently insert a padded tongue blade between the back molars if necessary.	
——	——	——	6. If teeth are present, brush carefully with toothbrush and paste. Remove dentures if present and use a toothette or gauze-padded tongue blade moistened with water or dilute mouthwash solution to gently cleanse gums, mucous membranes, and tongue. Clean the dentures before replacing.	
——	——	——	7. Use gauze-padded tongue blade or toothette dipped in mouthwash solution to rinse the oral cavity. If desired, insert the rubber tip of the irrigating syringe into the patient's mouth and rinse gently with a small amount of water. Position the patient's head to allow for return of water or use suction apparatus to remove water from the oral cavity.	
——	——	——	8. Apply lubricant to the patient's lips.	
——	——	——	9. Remove equipment and return the patient to a position of comfort. Remove your gloves. Raise side rail and lower bed.	
——	——	——	10. Perform hand hygiene.	

Skill Checklists to Accompany Fundamentals of Nursing:
The Art and Science of Nursing Care, 6th edition

Name _____   Date _____

Unit _____   Position _____

Instructor/Evaluator: _____   Position _____

SKILL 37-4
Applying and Removing Antiembolism Stockings

Goal: The stockings will be applied and removed with minimal discomfort to patient.

Excellent	Satisfactory	Needs Practice		Comments
___	___	___	1. Check the patient's identification band and ask the patient to state his or her name, if appropriate.	
___	___	___	2. Explain what you are going to do and the rationale for use of elastic stockings.	
___	___	___	3. Close curtains around bed and close door to room if possible.	
___	___	___	4. Perform hand hygiene.	
___	___	___	5. Assist the patient to the supine position. If the patient has been sitting or walking, have him or her lie down with legs and feet well elevated for at least 15 minutes before applying stockings.	
___	___	___	6. Expose the legs one at a time. Wash and dry legs, if necessary. Powder the leg lightly unless the patient has a breathing problem, dry skin, or sensitivity to the powder. If the skin is dry, a lotion may be used. Powders and lotions are not recommended by some manufacturers; check the package material for manufacturer specifications.	
___	___	___	7. Stand at the foot of the bed. Place a hand inside the stocking and grasp the heel area securely. Turn the stocking inside-out to the heel area, leaving the foot inside the stocking leg.	
___	___	___	8. With the heel pocket down, ease the foot of the stocking over the patient's foot and heel. Check that the patient's heel is centered in the heel pocket of the stocking.	
___	___	___	9. Using your fingers and thumbs, carefully grasp the edge of the stocking and pull it up smoothly over the patient's ankle and calf, toward the knee. Make sure it is distributed evenly.	
___	___	___	10. Pull forward slightly on the toe section. If the stocking has a toe window, make sure it is properly positioned. Adjust if necessary to ensure material is smooth.	

Excellent	Satisfactory	Needs Practice		Comments
——	——	——	11. If the stockings are knee-length, make sure each stocking top is 1 to 2 inches below the patella. Make sure the stocking does not roll down.	
——	——	——	12. If applying thigh-length stockings, continue the application. Flex the patient's leg. Stretch the stocking over the knee.	
——	——	——	13. Pull the stocking over the thigh until the top is 1 to 3 inches below the gluteal fold. Adjust the stocking as necessary to distribute the fabric evenly. Make sure the stocking does not roll down.	
——	——	——	14. Perform hand hygiene.	

Removing Stockings

To remove stocking, grasp top of stocking with your thumb and fingers and smoothly pull stocking off inside-out to heel. Support foot and ease stocking over it.

Skill Checklists to Accompany Fundamentals of Nursing:
The Art and Science of Nursing Care, 6th edition

Name _____   Date _____

Unit _____   Position _____

Instructor/Evaluator: _____   Position _____

Excellent	Satisfactory	Needs Practice	SKILL 37-5 **Making an Unoccupied Bed**	
			Goal: The bed linens will be changed without injury to the nurse or patient.	**Comments**
___	___	___	1. Assemble equipment and arrange on a bedside chair in the order in which items will be used.	
___	___	___	2. Perform hand hygiene.	
___	___	___	3. Adjust bed to high position and drop side rails.	
___	___	___	4. Disconnect call bell or any tubes from bed linens.	
___	___	___	5. Put on gloves if linens are soiled. Loosen all linen as you move around the bed, from the head of the bed on the far side to the head of the bed on the near side.	
___	___	___	6. Fold reusable linens, such as sheets, blankets, or spread, in place on the bed in fourths and hang them over a clean chair.	
___	___	___	7. **Snugly roll all the soiled linen inside the bottom sheet and place directly into the laundry hamper. Do not place on floor or furniture. Do not hold soiled linens against your uniform.**	
___	___	___	8. If possible, shift the mattress up to head of bed. If the mattress is soiled, clean and dry according to facility policy before applying new sheets.	
___	___	___	9. Remove your gloves. Place the bottom sheet with its center fold in the center of the bed. Open the sheet and fan-fold to the center.	
___	___	___	10. If using, place the drawsheet with its center fold in the center of the bed and positioned so it will be located under the patient's midsection. Open the drawsheet and fan-fold to the center of the mattress. If a protective pad is used, place it over the drawsheet in the proper area and open to the centerfold. Not all agencies use drawsheets routinely. The nurse may decide to use one.	

Excellent	Satisfactory	Needs Practice	SKILL 37-5 **Making an Unoccupied Bed** *(Continued)*	Comments
——	——	——	11. **For fitted bottom sheet:** Pull the bottom sheet over the corners at the head and foot of the mattress. Tuck the drawsheet securely under the mattress. **For a flat bottom sheet:** Corners are usually mitered. Grasp the side edge of the sheet about 18 inches down from the mattress top. Lay the sheet on top of the mattress to form a triangular, flat fold. Tuck the portion of the sheet that is hanging loose below the mattress under the mattress without pulling on the triangular fold. Pick up the top of the triangle fold and place it over the side of the mattress. Tuck this loose portion of the sheet under the mattress. Continue tucking the remaining bottom sheet and drawsheet securely under the mattress.	
——	——	——	12. Move to the other side of the bed to secure bottom linens. Pull the bottom sheet tightly and secure over the corners at the head and foot of the mattress. Pull the drawsheet tightly and tuck it securely under the mattress.	
——	——	——	13. Place the top sheet on the bed with its center fold in the center of the bed and with the hem even with the head of the mattress. Unfold the top sheet. Follow the same procedure with top blanket or spread, placing the upper edge about 6″ below the top of the sheet.	
——	——	——	14. Tuck the top sheet and blanket under the foot of the bed on the near side. Miter the corners.	
——	——	——	15. Fold the upper 6″ of the top sheet down over the spread and make a cuff.	
——	——	——	16. Move to the other side of the bed and follow the same procedure for securing top sheets under the foot of the bed and making a cuff.	
——	——	——	17. Place the pillows on the bed. Open each pillowcase in the same manner as you opened the other linens. Gather the pillowcase over one hand toward the closed end. Grasp the pillow with the hand inside the pillowcase. Keep a firm hold on the top of the pillow and pull the cover onto the pillow. Place the pillow at the head of the bed.	
——	——	——	18. Fan-fold or pie-fold the top linens.	
——	——	——	19. **Secure the signal device on the bed according to agency policy.**	
——	——	——	20. **Adjust bed to low position.**	
——	——	——	21. Dispose of soiled linen according to agency policy. Perform hand hygiene.	

Skill Checklists to Accompany Fundamentals of Nursing:
The Art and Science of Nursing Care, 6th edition

Name _____   Date _____

Unit _____   Position _____

Instructor/Evaluator: _____   Position _____

Excellent	Satisfactory	Needs Practice	SKILL 37-6 **Making an Occupied Bed**	Comments
			Goal: The bed linens are applied without injury to the patient or nurse.	
___	___	___	1. Identify the patient. Explain the procedure to the patient. Check the chart for limitations on the patient's physical activity.	
___	___	___	2. Perform hand hygiene.	
___	___	___	3. Assemble equipment and arrange on bedside chair in the order the items will be used.	
___	___	___	4. Close the door or curtain.	
___	___	___	5. Adjust bed to high position. Lower the side rail nearest you, leaving the opposite side rail up. Place bed in flat position unless contraindicated.	
___	___	___	6. Check bed linens for the patient's personal items. **Disconnect the call bell or any tubes/drains from bed linens.**	
___	___	___	7. Put on gloves if linens are soiled. Place a bath blanket over the patient. Have the patient hold onto the bath blanket while you reach under it and remove the top linens. Leave the top sheet in place if a bath blanket is not used. Fold the linen that is to be reused over the back of a chair. Discard soiled linen in a laundry bag or hamper. Keep soiled linen away from uniform.	
___	___	___	8. If possible and another person is available to assist, grasp the mattress securely and shift it up to the head of bed.	
___	___	___	9. Assist the patient to turn toward the opposite side of the bed, and reposition the pillow under patient's head.	
___	___	___	10. Loosen all bottom linens from head, foot, and side of bed.	
___	___	___	11. Fan-fold soiled linens as close to patient as possible.	
___	___	___	12. Remove your gloves, if used. Use clean linen and make the near side of the bed. Place the bottom sheet with its center fold in the center of the bed. Open the sheet and fan-fold to the center, positioning it under the old linens. Pull the bottom sheet over the corners at the head and foot of the mattress.	

Excellent	Satisfactory	Needs Practice		Comments
			## SKILL 37-6 ## Making an Occupied Bed *(Continued)*	
—	—	—	13. If using a drawsheet, place it with its center fold in the center of the bed and positioned so it will be located under the patient's midsection. Open the drawsheet and fan-fold to the center of the mattress. Tuck the drawsheet securely under the mattress. If a protective pad is used, place it over the drawsheet in the proper area and open to the centerfold. Not all agencies use drawsheets routinely. The nurse may decide to use one.	
—	—	—	14. Raise the side rail. Assist the patient to roll over the folded linen in the middle of the bed toward you. Reposition the pillow and bath blanket or top sheet. Move to the other side of the bed and lower the side rail.	
—	—	—	15. Put on clean gloves if linen is soiled. Loosen and remove all bottom linen. Place in a linen bag or hamper. Hold soiled linen away from your uniform. Remove gloves, if used.	
—	—	—	16. Ease clean linen from under the patient. Pull the bottom sheet taut and secure at the corners at the head and foot of the mattress. Pull the drawsheet tight and smooth. Tuck the drawsheet securely under the mattress.	
—	—	—	17. Assist the patient to turn back to the center of bed. If the pillowcase is soiled with blood or body fluids, put on unsterile gloves. Remove the pillow and change the pillowcase. Open each pillowcase in the same manner as you opened other linens. Gather the pillowcase over one hand toward the closed end. Grasp the pillow with the hand inside the pillowcase. Keep a firm hold on the top of the pillow and pull the cover onto the pillow. Place the pillow under the patient's head. Remove gloves, if worn.	
—	—	—	18. Apply top linen, sheet and blanket if desired, so that it is centered. Fold the top linens over at the patient's shoulders to make a cuff. Have the patient hold onto top linen and remove the bath blanket from underneath.	
—	—	—	19. Secure top linens under the foot of the mattress and miter corners. Loosen top linens over the patient's feet by grasping them in the area of the feet and pulling gently toward the foot of bed.	
—	—	—	20. **Raise the side rail. Lower bed height and adjust the head of bed to a comfortable position. Reattach the call bell.**	
—	—	—	21. Dispose of soiled linens according to agency policy. Perform hand hygiene.	

Skill Checklists to Accompany Fundamentals of Nursing:
The Art and Science of Nursing Care, 6th edition

Name _____ Date _____

Unit _____ Position _____

Instructor/Evaluator: _____ Position _____

SKILL 38-1

Cleaning a Wound and Applying a Dry, Sterile Dressing

Goal: The wound is cleaned and protected with a dressing without contaminating the wound area, without causing trauma to the wound, and without causing the patient to experience pain or discomfort.

Excellent	Satisfactory	Needs Practice		Comments
___	___	___	1. Review the physician's order for wound care or the nursing plan of care related to wound care.	
___	___	___	2. Gather the necessary supplies.	
___	___	___	3. Identify the patient.	
___	___	___	4. Explain the procedure to the patient.	
___	___	___	5. Assess the patient for possible need for nonpharmacologic pain-reducing interventions or analgesic medication prior to wound care dressing change. Administer appropriate analgesic, consulting physician's orders, and allow enough time for analgesic to achieve its effectiveness.	
___	___	___	6. Perform hand hygiene.	
___	___	___	7. Close the room door or curtains. Place the bed at an appropriate and comfortable working height.	
___	___	___	8. Place a waste receptacle or bag at a convenient location for use during the procedure.	
___	___	___	9. Assist the patient to a comfortable position that provides easy access to the wound area. Use the bath blanket to cover any exposed area other than the wound. If necessary, place the waterproof pad under the wound site.	
___	___	___	10. Check the position of drains, tubes, or other adjuncts before removing the dressing. Put on clean, disposable gloves and loosen the tape on the old dressings. If necessary, use an adhesive remover to help remove the tape.	
___	___	___	11. Carefully remove the soiled dressings. If any part of the dressing sticks to the underlying skin, use small amounts of sterile saline to help loosen and remove. Do not reach over the wound.	
___	___	___	12. After removing the dressing, note the presence, amount, type, color, and odor of any drainage on the dressings. Place soiled dressings in the appropriate waste receptacle. Remove your gloves and dispose of them in an appropriate waste receptacle.	

SKILL 38-1
Cleaning a Wound and Applying a Dry, Sterile Dressing (Continued)

Excellent	Satisfactory	Needs Practice		Comments
——	——	——	13. Inspect the wound site for size, appearance, and drainage. Assess if any pain is present. Check the sutures, Steri-Strips, staples, and drains or tubes. Note any problems to include in your documentation.	
——	——	——	14. **Using sterile technique, prepare a sterile work area and open the needed supplies.**	
——	——	——	15. Open the sterile cleaning solution. Depending on the amount of cleaning needed, the solution might be poured directly over gauze sponges for small cleaning jobs or over a container or into a basin for more complex or larger cleaning.	
——	——	——	16. Put on sterile gloves.	
——	——	——	17. Clean the wound. If needed, use sterile forceps to clean the area. **Clean the wound from top to bottom and from the center to the outside. Following this pattern, use a new gauze for each wipe, placing the used gauze in the waste receptacle. Do not touch any surface with the gloves or forceps.**	
——	——	——	18. **If a drain is in use, clean around the drain using a circular motion. Wipe from the center toward the outside. Use the gauze a single time and then dispose of it.**	
——	——	——	19. Once the wound is cleansed, dry the area using a gauze sponge in the same manner. Apply ointment or any other treatments if ordered.	
——	——	——	20. Apply a layer of dry sterile dressing over the wound. Forceps may be used to apply the dressing.	
——	——	——	21. Place a second layer of gauze over the wound site.	
——	——	——	22. Apply a Surgi-Pad or ABD dressing over the gauze at the site as the outermost layer of the dressing.	
——	——	——	23. Remove and discard sterile gloves. Apply tape or tie tapes to secure the dressings.	
——	——	——	24. After securing the dressing, label dressing with date and time. Remove all remaining equipment, place the patient in a comfortable position with side rails up and bed in the lowest position. Perform hand hygiene.	
——	——	——	25. Check all wound dressings every shift. More frequent checks may be needed if the wound is more complex or dressings become saturated quickly.	

Skill Checklists to Accompany Fundamentals of Nursing:
The Art and Science of Nursing Care, 6th edition

Name _____   Date _____

Unit _____   Position _____

Instructor/Evaluator: _____   Position _____

Excellent	Satisfactory	Needs Practice	SKILL 38-2 **Applying a Saline-Moistened Dressing**	Comments
			Goal: The procedure is accomplished without contaminating the wound area, without causing trauma to the wound, and without causing the patient to experience pain or discomfort.	
___	___	___	1. Review the physician's order and/or nursing care plan for the application of a saline-moistened dressing.	
___	___	___	2. Gather the necessary supplies.	
___	___	___	3. Identify the patient.	
___	___	___	4. Explain the procedure to the patient.	
___	___	___	5. Assess the patient for possible need for nonpharmacologic pain-reducing interventions or analgesic medication prior to wound care dressing change. Administer appropriate analgesic, consulting physician's orders, and allow enough time for analgesic to achieve its effectiveness before beginning procedure.	
___	___	___	6. Perform hand hygiene.	
___	___	___	7. Close the room door or curtains. Place the bed at a comfortable working height.	
___	___	___	8. Place a waste receptacle or bag at a convenient location for use during procedure.	
___	___	___	9. Assist the patient to a comfortable position that provides easy access to the wound area. Position the patient so the irrigation solution will flow from the clean end of the wound toward the dirtier end, if wound irrigation is necessary (see Skill 38-3 for irrigation techniques). Expose the area and drape the patient with the bath blanket if needed. Put the waterproof pad under the wound area to protect the bed.	
___	___	___	10. Put on personal protective equipment as appropriate.	
___	___	___	11. Put on clean disposable gloves and gently remove the soiled dressings. If the dressing adheres to the underlying tissues, moisten it with saline to loosen it.	
___	___	___	12. After removing the dressing, note the presence, amount, type, color, and odor of any drainage on the dressings. Place soiled dressings in the appropriate waste receptacle.	

Applying a Saline-Moistened Dressing (Continued)

Excellent	Satisfactory	Needs Practice		Comments
——	——	——	13. Assess the wound for appearance, stage, the presence of eschar, granulation tissue, epithelialization, undermining, tunneling, necrosis, sinus tract, and drainage. Assess the appearance of the surrounding tissue. Measure the wound.	
——	——	——	14. Remove your gloves and put them in the receptacle.	
——	——	——	15. Using sterile technique, open the supplies and dressings. Place the fine-mesh gauze into the basin and pour the ordered solution over the mesh to saturate it.	
——	——	——	16. Put on the sterile gloves.	
——	——	——	17. Clean the wound. If needed, use sterile forceps to clean the area. **Clean the wound from top to bottom and from the center to the outside. Following this pattern, use a new gauze for each wipe, placing the used gauze in the waste receptacle. Do not touch any surface with the gloves or forceps.** Irrigate the wound, if needed (see Skill 38-3).	
——	——	——	18. Dry the surrounding skin with sterile gauze dressings.	
——	——	——	19. Squeeze excess fluid from the gauze dressing. Unfold and fluff the dressing.	
——	——	——	20. Gently press to loosely pack the moistened gauze into the wound. If necessary, use the forceps or cotton-tipped applicators to press the gauze into all wound surfaces.	
——	——	——	21. Apply several dry, sterile gauze pads over the wet gauze.	
——	——	——	22. Place the ABD pad over the gauze.	
——	——	——	23. Remove and discard your sterile gloves. Apply a skin protectant to the surrounding skin if needed. Apply tape or tie tapes to secure the dressings.	
——	——	——	24. After securing the dressing, remove all remaining equipment, place the patient in a position of comfort with side rails up and the bed in the lowest position, and perform hand hygiene.	
——	——	——	25. Check all wound dressings every shift. You might need to check more frequently if a wound is more complex or dressings become saturated more frequently.	

Skill Checklists to Accompany Fundamentals of Nursing:
The Art and Science of Nursing Care, 6th edition

Name _____   Date _____

Unit _____   Position _____

Instructor/Evaluator: _____   Position _____

Excellent	Satisfactory	Needs Practice	SKILL 38-3 **Performing a Sterile Irrigation of a Wound**	Comments
			Goal: The wound is cleaned without contamination or trauma and without causing the patient to experience pain or discomfort.	
____	____	____	1. Review the physician's order for wound care or the nursing plan of care related to wound care.	
____	____	____	2. Gather the necessary supplies.	
____	____	____	3. Identify the patient.	
____	____	____	4. Explain the procedure to the patient.	
____	____	____	5. Assess the patient for possible need for nonpharmacologic pain-reducing interventions or analgesic medication prior to wound care dressing change. Administer appropriate analgesic, consulting physician's orders, and allow enough time for analgesic to achieve its effectiveness.	
____	____	____	6. Perform hand hygiene.	
____	____	____	7. Close the room door or curtains. Place the bed at a comfortable working height.	
____	____	____	8. Have the disposal bag or waste receptacle within easy reach prior to the irrigation for soiled dressing disposal.	
____	____	____	9. Assist the patient to a comfortable position that provides easy access to the wound area. **Position the patient so that the irrigation solution will flow from the clean to dirty end of the wound.** Expose the area and drape the patient with a bath blanket if needed. Put the waterproof pad under the wound area.	
____	____	____	10. Put on a gown, mask, and eye protection.	
____	____	____	11. Put on clean disposable gloves and remove the soiled dressings.	
____	____	____	12. Assess the wound for size, appearance, and drainage on the dressing. Assess the appearance of the surrounding tissue.	
____	____	____	13. Discard the dressings in the receptacle. Remove gloves and put them in the receptacle.	
____	____	____	14. **Using sterile technique, prepare a sterile field and add all the sterile supplies needed for the procedure to the field. Pour warmed sterile irrigating solution into the sterile container.**	

74

Performing a Sterile Irrigation of a Wound *(Continued)*

Excellent	Satisfactory	Needs Practice		Comments
——	——	——	15. Put on sterile gloves.	
——	——	——	16. Position the sterile basin below the wound to collect the irrigation fluid.	
——	——	——	17. Fill the irrigation syringe with solution. **Using your nondominant hand, gently apply pressure to the basin against the skin below the wound to form a seal with the skin.**	
——	——	——	18. **Gently direct a stream of solution into the wound. Keep the tip of the syringe at least 1 inch above the upper tip of the wound. When using a catheter tip, insert it gently into the wound until it meets resistance. Gently flush all wound areas.**	
——	——	——	19. Watch for the solution to flow smoothly and evenly. When the solution from the wound flows out clear, discontinue irrigation.	
——	——	——	20. Dry the surrounding skin with a sterile gauze sponge.	
——	——	——	21. Apply a new sterile dressing to the wound (see Skill 38-1).	
——	——	——	22. Remove gloves and dispose of them properly. Apply a skin protectant to the surrounding skin if needed. Apply tie straps or tape as needed to secure the dressing. Remove other protective equipment and dispose in bedside waste receptacle container or bag.	
——	——	——	23. Return the bed to the lowest position while making the patient comfortable and raising the side rails as needed.	
——	——	——	24. Remove any remaining personal protective equipment and the waste receptacle out of the patient's room and dispose of it properly. If any irrigating solution remains in the bottle, recap the bottle and note on the bottle the date and time it was opened.	
——	——	——	25. Perform hand hygiene.	
——	——	——	26. Check all wound dressings every shift. You might need to check more frequently if a wound is more complex or dressings become saturated more frequently.	

Skill Checklists to Accompany Fundamentals of Nursing:
The Art and Science of Nursing Care, 6th edition

Name _____   Date _____

Unit _____   Position _____

Instructor/Evaluator: _____   Position _____

Excellent	Satisfactory	Needs Practice	SKILL 38-4 **Caring for a Jackson-Pratt Drain**	
			Goal: The drain is patent and intact.	**Comments**
___	___	___	1. Review the physician's order for drain and site care or the nursing plan of care related to drain care.	
___	___	___	2. Gather the necessary supplies.	
___	___	___	3. Identify the patient.	
___	___	___	4. Assess the patient for possible need for nonpharmacologic pain-reducing interventions or analgesic medication prior to wound care dressing change. Administer appropriate analgesic, consulting physician's orders, and allow enough time for analgesic to achieve its effectiveness.	
___	___	___	5. Perform hand hygiene.	
___	___	___	6. Close the room door or curtains. Place the bed at an appropriate and comfortable working height.	
___	___	___	7. Assist the patient to a comfortable position that provides easy access to the drain area. Use the bath blanket to cover any exposed area other than the drain. Place the waterproof pad under the drain site.	
___	___	___	8. Put on clean gloves; put on mask or face shield, if indicated.	
___	___	___	9. Place the graduated collection container under the outlet valve of the drain. Without contaminating the outlet valve, pull the cap off. The chamber will expand completely as it draws in air. **Empty the chamber's contents completely into the container. Use the alcohol pad to clean the chamber's spout and cap. Fully compress the chamber with one hand and replace the plug with your other hand.**	
___	___	___	10. Check the patency of the equipment. Make sure the tubing is free from twists and kinks.	
___	___	___	11. Secure the Jackson-Pratt drain to the patient's gown below the wound with a safety pin, making sure that there is no tension on the tubing.	
___	___	___	12. Carefully measure and record the character, color, and amount of the drainage. Discard the drainage according to facility policy.	

Caring for a Jackson-Pratt Drain *(Continued)*

Excellent	Satisfactory	Needs Practice		Comments
——	——	——	13. If the drain site has a dressing, redress the site.	
——	——	——	14. If the drain site is open to air, observe the sutures that secure the drain to the skin. Look for signs of pulling, tearing, swelling, or infection of the surrounding skin.	
——	——	——	15. Gently clean the sutures with the gauze pad soaked in normal saline. Dry with a new gauze pad. Apply skin protectant to the surrounding skin if needed.	
——	——	——	16. Remove gloves and all remaining equipment, place the patient in a position of comfort with side rails up and bed in the lowest position, and perform hand hygiene.	

Name _____ Date _____

Unit _____ Position _____

Instructor/Evaluator: _____ Position _____

Excellent	Satisfactory	Needs Practice	SKILL 38-5 **Caring for a Hemovac Drain**	
			Goal: The drain is patent and intact.	**Comments**
___	___	___	1. Review the physician's order for drain and site care or the nursing plan of care related to drain care.	
___	___	___	2. Gather the necessary supplies.	
___	___	___	3. Identify the patient.	
___	___	___	4. Explain the procedure to the patient.	
___	___	___	5. Assess the patient for possible need for nonpharmacologic pain-reducing interventions or analgesic medication prior to wound care dressing change. Administer appropriate analgesic, consulting physician's orders, and allow enough time for analgesic to achieve its effectiveness.	
___	___	___	6. Perform hand hygiene.	
___	___	___	7. Close the room door or curtains. Place the bed at an appropriate and comfortable working height.	
___	___	___	8. Assist the patient to a comfortable position that provides easy access to the drain area. Use the bath blanket to cover any exposed area other than the drain. Place the waterproof pad under the drain site.	
___	___	___	9. Put on clean gloves and other personal protective equipment, such as mask or face shield, as necessary.	
___	___	___	10. Place the graduated collection container under the pouring spout of the drain. Without contaminating the outlet valve, uncap the valve. The chamber will expand completely as it draws in air. Empty the chamber's contents completely into the container. Use the alcohol pad to clean the chamber's spout and cap. **Fully compress the chamber by pushing the top and bottom together with your hands. Keep the device tightly compressed while you reinsert the plug.**	
___	___	___	11. Check the patency of the equipment. Make sure the tubing is free from twists and kinks.	
___	___	___	12. Secure the Hemovac drain to the patient's gown below the wound with pins, making sure that there is no tension on the tubing.	

Excellent	Satisfactory	Needs Practice	SKILL 38-5 **Caring for a Hemovac Drain** *(Continued)*	
				Comments
——	——	——	13. Carefully measure and record the character, color, and amount of the drainage. Discard the drainage according to facility policy.	
——	——	——	14. If the drain site has a dressing, redress the site. Assess the patient for possible need for pain/analgesic medication prior to dressing change.	
——	——	——	15. If the drain site is open to air, observe the sutures that secure the drain to the skin. Look for signs of pulling, tearing, swelling, or infection of the surrounding skin.	
——	——	——	16. Gently clean the sutures with the gauze pad soaked in normal saline. Dry with a new gauze pad.	
——	——	——	17. Remove gloves and all remaining equipment, place the patient in a position of comfort with side rails up and bed in the lowest position, and perform hand hygiene.	

Skill Checklists to Accompany Fundamentals of Nursing:
The Art and Science of Nursing Care, 6th edition

Name _____   Date _____

Unit _____   Position _____

Instructor/Evaluator: _____   Position _____

SKILL 38-6

Collecting a Wound Culture

Goal: The culture is obtained without evidence of contamination, without exposing the patient to additional pathogens and without causing discomfort for the patient.

Excellent	Satisfactory	Needs Practice		Comments
___	___	___	1. Review the physician's order for obtaining a wound culture.	
___	___	___	2. Gather the necessary supplies.	
___	___	___	3. Identify the patient.	
___	___	___	4. Explain the procedure to the patient.	
___	___	___	5. Perform hand hygiene.	
___	___	___	6. Close the room door or curtains. Place the bed at an appropriate and comfortable working height.	
___	___	___	7. Place an appropriate waste receptacle within easy reach for use during the procedure.	
___	___	___	8. Assist the patient to a comfortable position that provides easy access to the wound. If necessary, drape the patient with the bath blanket to expose only the wound area. Check the culture label again against the patient's identification bracelet.	
___	___	___	9. Put on the clean, disposable gloves to remove any dressings. Loosen the tape and old dressings. Do not reach over the wound. Remove the dressing and dispose of it in the receptacle. Assess the wound and the characteristics of any drainage. Remove gloves and dispose of them.	
___	___	___	10. Set up a sterile field with supplies if necessary. Put on sterile gloves and clean the wound according to facility policies and procedures. Remove the sterile gloves.	
___	___	___	11. Put on clean gloves. Twist the cap to loosen the swab on the Culturette tube, or open the separate swab and remove the cap from the culture tube. **Keep the swab and inside of the culture tube sterile.**	
___	___	___	12. Put on a clean glove or new sterile glove, if necessary.	
___	___	___	13. **Carefully insert the swab into the wound and gently roll the swab to obtain a sample. Use another swab if collecting a specimen from another site.**	

Collecting a Wound Culture (Continued)

Excellent	Satisfactory	Needs Practice		Comments
——	——	——	14. Place the swab back in the culture tube. **Do not touch the outside of the tube with the swab.** Secure the cap. Some Culturette tubes have an ampule of medium at the bottom of the tube. It might be necessary to crush this ampule to activate. Follow the manufacturer's instructions for use.	
——	——	——	15. Remove gloves and discard them accordingly.	
——	——	——	16. Put on sterile gloves and replace the dressing as needed following the appropriate procedure.	
——	——	——	17. Remove gloves and perform hand hygiene. Remove any equipment and leave the patient comfortable, with the side rails up and the bed in the lowest position.	
——	——	——	18. Label the specimen according to your institution's guidelines and send it to the laboratory in a biohazard bag.	

Skill Checklists to Accompany Fundamentals of Nursing:
The Art and Science of Nursing Care, 6th edition

Name _____   Date _____

Unit _____   Position _____

Instructor/Evaluator: _____   Position _____

SKILL 38-7

Applying a Wound Vacuum-Assisted Closure

Goal: The therapy is accomplished without contaminating the wound area, without causing trauma to the wound, and without causing the patient to experience pain or discomfort.

Excellent	Satisfactory	Needs Practice		Comments
____	____	____	1. Review the physician's order for the application of wound VAC therapy, including the ordered setting for the negative pressure.	
____	____	____	2. Gather the necessary supplies.	
____	____	____	3. Identify the patient.	
____	____	____	4. Explain the procedure.	
____	____	____	5. Assess the patient for possible need for nonpharmacologic pain-reducing interventions or analgesic medication prior to wound care dressing change. Administer appropriate analgesic, consulting physician's orders, and allow enough time for analgesic to achieve its effectiveness before beginning procedure.	
____	____	____	6. Perform hand hygiene.	
____	____	____	7. Close the room door or curtains. Place the bed in a comfortable working height.	
____	____	____	8. Assist the patient to a comfortable position that provides easy access to the wound area. Position the patient so the irrigation solution will flow from the clean end of the wound toward the dirty end. Expose the area and drape the patient with a bath blanket if needed. Put a waterproof pad under the wound area.	
____	____	____	9. Have the disposal bag or waste receptacle within easy reach for use during the procedure.	
____	____	____	10. Assemble the VAC device according to the manufacturer's instructions. Set the negative pressure according to the physician's order (25 to 200 mm Hg).	
____	____	____	11. Using sterile technique, prepare a sterile field and add all the sterile supplies needed for the procedure to the field. Pour warmed sterile irrigating solution into the sterile container.	
____	____	____	12. Put on a gown, mask, and eye protection.	
____	____	____	13. Put on clean disposable gloves and remove the soiled dressings.	

Excellent	Satisfactory	Needs Practice	SKILL 38-7 **Applying a Wound Vacuum-Assisted Closure** *(Continued)*	Comments
——	——	——	14. Assess the wound for appearance and drainage. Assess the appearance of the surrounding tissue.	
——	——	——	15. Discard the dressings in the receptacle. Remove your gloves and put them in the receptacle.	
——	——	——	16. Put on sterile gloves. Using sterile technique, irrigate the wound (see Skill 38-3).	
——	——	——	17. Clean the area around the skin with normal saline. Dry the surrounding skin with a sterile gauze sponge.	
——	——	——	18. **Wipe intact skin around the wound with a skin protectant wipe and allow it to dry well.**	
——	——	——	19. Remove gloves if they become contaminated and discard them into the receptacle.	
——	——	——	20. Put on a new pair of sterile gloves. **Using sterile scissors, cut the foam to the shape and measurement of the wound.** More than one piece of foam may be necessary if the first piece is cut too small. **Carefully place the foam in the wound.**	
——	——	——	21. **Place the fenestrated tubing into the center of the foam. There should be foam between the tubing and the base of the wound and foam over the top of the tubing.**	
——	——	——	22. **Cover the foam and tubing with the transparent occlusive air-permeable dressing, leaving at least a 2-inch margin on the intact skin around the wound.**	
——	——	——	23. Connect the free end of the fenestrated tubing to the tubing that is connected to the evacuation canister.	
——	——	——	24. Remove and discard gloves. Turn on the vacuum unit. **Observe the shrinking of the transparent dressing to the foam and skin.**	
——	——	——	25. Lower the bed and make sure the patient is comfortable.	
——	——	——	26. Perform hand hygiene.	
——	——	——	27. Dispose of used supplies and equipment according to facility policy.	
——	——	——	28. Check all wound dressings every shift.	

Skill Checklists to Accompany Fundamentals of Nursing:
The Art and Science of Nursing Care, 6th edition

Name _____ Date _____

Unit _____ Position _____

Instructor/Evaluator: _____ Position _____

SKILL 38-8

Applying an External Heating Device: Aquathermia Pad and Hot Water Bag

Goal: The patient experiences increased comfort; the patient experiences decreased muscle spasms; the patient exhibits improved wound healing; the patient demonstrates a reduction in inflammation; and the patient remains free of injury.

Excellent	Satisfactory	Needs Practice		Comments
___	___	___	1. Review the physician's order for the application of heat therapy, including frequency, type of therapy, body area to be treated, and length of time for the application.	
___	___	___	2. Gather the necessary supplies.	
___	___	___	3. Identify the patient.	
___	___	___	4. Explain the procedure.	
___	___	___	5. Assess the condition of the skin where the heat is to be applied.	
___	___	___	6. Perform hand hygiene.	
___	___	___	7. Close the room door or curtains. Place the bed at a comfortable working height.	
___	___	___	8. Assist the patient to a comfortable position that provides easy access to the area to be treated. Expose the area and drape the patient with a bath blanket if needed. Put a waterproof pad under the wound area to protect the bed, if necessary.	
___	___	___	9. Check that the water is at the appropriate level. Fill the control unit two-thirds full with distilled water, or to the fill mark, if necessary. Check the temperature setting on the unit to ensure it is within the safe range.	
___	___	___	10. Check for leaks and tilt the unit in several directions.	
___	___	___	11. Plug in the unit and warm the pad before use. Cover the pad with an absorbent cloth. Apply the heat source to the prescribed area. Secure with gauze bandage or tape.	
___	___	___	12. **Assess the condition of the skin and the patient's response to the heat at frequent intervals, according to facility policy. Do not exceed the prescribed length of time for the application of heat.**	
___	___	___	13. Remove after the prescribed amount of time. Perform hand hygiene.	

84

Skill Checklists to Accompany Fundamentals of Nursing:
The Art and Science of Nursing Care, 6th edition

Name _____   Date _____

Unit _____   Position _____

Instructor/Evaluator: _____   Position _____

Excellent	Satisfactory	Needs Practice	SKILL 38-9 **Applying a Warm Sterile Compress to an Open Wound**	Comments
			Goal: The patient shows signs, such as decreased inflammation, decreased muscle spasms, or decreased pain, that indicate problems have been relieved.	
___	___	___	1. Review the physician's order.	
___	___	___	2. Gather the necessary supplies.	
___	___	___	3. Identify the patient.	
___	___	___	4. Explain the procedure.	
___	___	___	5. Assess the patient for the possible need for nonpharmacologic pain-reducing interventions or analgesic medication prior to wound care dressing change. Administer appropriate analgesic, consulting physician's orders, and allow enough time for analgesic to achieve its effectiveness before beginning procedure.	
___	___	___	6. Perform hand hygiene.	
___	___	___	7. Close the room door or curtains. Place the bed at a comfortable working height.	
___	___	___	8. Assist the patient to a comfortable position that provides easy access to the wound area. Expose the area and drape the patient with a bath blanket if needed. Put the waterproof pad under the wound area.	
___	___	___	9. Have the disposal bag or waste receptacle within easy reach for use during the procedure.	
___	___	___	10. Prepare the external heating pad or Aquathermia pad if one is being used.	
___	___	___	11. Using sterile technique, prepare a working field and open all sterile packaging, dressings, and the warmed solution. Pour the solution into the sterile container and drop the sterile gauze for the compress into the solution.	
___	___	___	12. Put on clean disposable gloves and remove any old dressing in place. Discard the old dressing in the appropriate receptacle. Remove your gloves and discard them.	
___	___	___	13. Assess the wound site and surrounding tissues. Look for inflammation, drainage, skin color, ecchymosis, and odor.	
___	___	___	14. Put on sterile gloves, following proper procedure.	

Excellent	Satisfactory	Needs Practice	SKILL 38-9 **Applying a Warm Sterile Compress to an Open Wound** *(Continued)*	
				Comments
——	——	——	15. Retrieve the sterile compress from the warmed solution, squeezing out any excess moisture. Apply the compress by gently and carefully molding it around the wound site. Ask the patient if the application feels too hot.	
——	——	——	16. **Cover the site with a single layer of gauze and with a clean dry bath towel;** secure in place if necessary.	
——	——	——	17. Place the Aquathermia or heating device, if used, over the towel.	
——	——	——	18. Remove sterile gloves and discard them appropriately. Perform hand hygiene.	
——	——	——	19. **Monitor the time the compress is in place to prevent burns or skin damage. Monitor the condition of the patient's skin and the patient's response at frequent intervals.**	
——	——	——	20. After the prescribed time for the treatment (up to 30 minutes), remove the external heating device (if used) and put on sterile gloves.	
——	——	——	21. Carefully remove the compress while assessing the skin condition around the wound site and observing the patient's response to the heat application. Note any wound changes.	
——	——	——	22. Apply a new dry sterile dressing to the wound, following proper procedure.	
——	——	——	23. Remove gloves. Place the patient in a comfortable position. Lower the bed. Dispose of any other supplies appropriately.	
——	——	——	24. Perform hand hygiene.	

Skill Checklists to Accompany Fundamentals of Nursing:
The Art and Science of Nursing Care, 6th edition

Name _____   Date _____

Unit _____   Position _____

Instructor/Evaluator: _____   Position _____

Excellent	Satisfactory	Needs Practice	SKILL 39-1 **Providing Range-of-Motion Exercises**	
			Goal: The patient maintains joint mobility.	**Comments**
____	____	____	1. Review the physician's orders and nursing plan of care for patient activity. Identify any movement limitations.	
____	____	____	2. Identify the patient. Explain the procedure to the patient.	
____	____	____	3. Perform hand hygiene and put on gloves, if necessary.	
____	____	____	4. Close the room door or curtains. Place the bed at an appropriate and comfortable working height. Adjust the head of the bed to a flat position or as low as the patient can tolerate.	
____	____	____	5. Stand on the side of the bed where the joints are to be exercised. Lower side rail on that side, if in place. Uncover only the limb to be used during the exercise.	
____	____	____	6. Perform the exercises slowly and gently, providing support by holding the areas proximal and distal to the joint. Repeat each exercise two to five times, moving each joint in a smooth and rhythmic manner. **Stop movement if the patient complains of pain or if you meet resistance.**	
____	____	____	7. **While performing the exercises, begin at the head and move down one side of the body at a time.**	
____	____	____	8. Move the chin down to rest on the chest. Return the head to a normal upright position. Tilt the head as far as possible toward each shoulder.	
____	____	____	9. Move the head from side to side, bringing the chin toward each shoulder.	
____	____	____	10. Start with the arm at the patient's side and lift the arm forward to above the head. Return the arm to the starting position at the side of the body.	
____	____	____	11. With the arm back at the patient's side, move the arm laterally to an upright position above the head, and then return to the original position. Move the arm across the body as far as possible.	

Excellent	Satisfactory	Needs Practice	SKILL 39-1 **Providing Range-of-Motion Exercises** (*Continued*)	Comments
——	——	——	12. Raise the arm at the side until the upper arm is in line with the shoulder. Bend the elbow at a 90-degree angle and move the forearm upward and downward, then return the arm to the side.	
——	——	——	13. Bend the elbow and move the lower arm and hand upward toward the shoulder. Return the lower arm and hand to the original position while straightening the elbow.	
——	——	——	14. Rotate the lower arm and hand so the palm is up. Rotate the lower arm and hand so the palm of the hand is down.	
——	——	——	15. Move the hand downward toward the inner aspect of the forearm. Return the hand to a neutral position even with the forearm. Then move the dorsal portion of the hand backward as far as possible.	
——	——	——	16. Bend the fingers to make a fist, and then straighten them out. Spread the fingers apart and return them back together. Touch the thumb to each finger on the hand.	
——	——	——	17. Extend the leg and lift it upward. Return the leg to the original position beside the other leg.	
——	——	——	18. Lift the leg laterally away from the patient's body. Return the leg back toward the other leg and try to extend it beyond the midline.	
——	——	——	19. Turn the foot and leg toward the other leg to rotate it internally. Turn the foot and leg outward away from the other leg to rotate it externally.	
——	——	——	20. Bend the leg and bring the heel toward the back of the leg. Return the leg to a straight position.	
——	——	——	21. At the ankle, move the foot up and back until the toes are upright. Move the foot with the toes pointing downward.	
——	——	——	22. Turn the sole of the foot toward the midline. Turn the sole of the foot outward.	
——	——	——	23. Curl the toes downward, and then straighten them out. Spread the toes apart and bring them together.	
——	——	——	24. Repeat these exercises on the other side of the body. Encourage the patient to do as many of these exercises by himself or herself as possible.	
——	——	——	25. When finished, make sure the patient is comfortable, with the side rails up and the bed in the lowest position.	
——	——	——	26. Remove gloves if used and perform hand hygiene.	

Skill Checklists to Accompany Fundamentals of Nursing:
The Art and Science of Nursing Care, 6th edition

Name _____   Date _____

Unit _____   Position _____

Instructor/Evaluator: _____   Position _____

Excellent	Satisfactory	Needs Practice	SKILL 39-2 **Assisting a Patient With Turning in Bed**	
			Goal: The activity takes place without injury to patient or nurse.	**Comments**
——	——	——	1. Review the physician's orders and nursing plan of care for patient activity. Identify any movement limitations and the ability of the patient to assist with turning. Consult patient handling algorithm, if available, to plan appropriate approach to moving the patient.	
——	——	——	2. Gather any positioning aids or supports, if necessary.	
——	——	——	3. Identify the patient. Explain the procedure to the patient.	
——	——	——	4. Perform hand hygiene and put on gloves, if necessary.	
——	——	——	5. Close the room door or curtains. Place the bed at an appropriate and comfortable working height.	
——	——	——	6. Adjust the head of the bed to a flat position or as low as the patient can tolerate. Place pillows, wedges, or any other supports to be used for positioning within easy reach.	
——	——	——	7. Lower the side rail nearest you if it has been raised. If not already in place, position a friction-reducing sheet or drawsheet under the patient.	
——	——	——	8. Using the friction-reducing sheet or drawsheet, move the patient to the edge of the bed, opposite the side to which he or she will be turned. Raise side rail and move to the opposite side of the bed.	
——	——	——	9. Stand on the side of the bed toward which the patient is turning. Lower the side rail nearest you.	
——	——	——	10. **Place the patient's arms across his or her chest and cross his or her far leg over the leg nearest you.**	
——	——	——	11. Stand opposite the patient's center with your feet spread about shoulder width and with one foot ahead of the other. **Tighten your gluteal and abdominal muscles and flex your knees. Use your leg muscles to do the pulling.**	
——	——	——	12. If available, activate the bed mechanism to inflate the side of the bed opposite from where you are standing.	

Excellent	Satisfactory	Needs Practice		Comments
			SKILL 39-2 **Assisting a Patient With Turning in Bed** *(Continued)*	

Excellent	Satisfactory	Needs Practice		Comments
___	___	___	13. Position your hands on the patient's far shoulder and hip, and roll the patient toward you, or you may use the friction-reducing sheet or drawsheet to gently pull the patient over on his or her side.	
___	___	___	14. Use a pillow or other support behind the patient's back. Pull the shoulder blade forward and out from under the patient.	
___	___	___	15. Make the patient comfortable and position in proper alignment, using pillows or other supports under the leg and arm as needed. Readjust the pillow under the patient's head. Elevate the head of the bed as needed for comfort.	
___	___	___	16. Place the bed in the lowest position, with the side rails up. Make sure the call bell and other necessary items are within easy reach.	
___	___	___	17. Perform hand hygiene.	

Skill Checklists to Accompany Fundamentals of Nursing:
The Art and Science of Nursing Care, 6th edition

Name _____   Date _____

Unit _____   Position _____

Instructor/Evaluator: _____   Position _____

SKILL 39-3

Moving a Patient Up in Bed With the Assistance of Another Nurse

Goal: The patient remains free from injury and maintains proper body alignment.

Excellent	Satisfactory	Needs Practice		Comments
___	___	___	1. Review the medical record and nursing plan of care for conditions that may influence the patient's ability to move or to be positioned. Assess for tubes, intravenous lines, incisions, or equipment that may alter the positioning procedure. Identify any movement limitations. Consult patient handling algorithm, if available, to plan appropriate approach to moving the patient.	
___	___	___	2. Identify the patient. Explain the procedure to the patient.	
___	___	___	3. Perform hand hygiene and put on gloves, if necessary.	
___	___	___	4. Close the room door or curtains. Place the bed at an appropriate and comfortable working height. Adjust the head of the bed to a flat position or as low as the patient can tolerate. Placing the bed in slight Trendelenburg position aids movement, if the patient is able to tolerate it.	
___	___	___	5. Remove all pillows from under the patient. Leave one at the head of the bed, leaning upright against the headboard.	
___	___	___	6. Position at least one nurse on either side of the bed, and lower both side rails.	
___	___	___	7. If a friction-reducing sheet or drawsheet is not in place under the patient, place one under the patient's midsection.	
___	___	___	8. Ask the patient (if able) to bend his or her legs and put his or her feet flat on the bed to assist with the movement.	
___	___	___	9. **Have the patient fold the arms across the chest. Have the patient (if able) lift the head with chin on chest.**	
___	___	___	10. Position yourself at the patient's midsection with your feet spread shoulder width apart and one foot slightly in front of the other.	
___	___	___	11. If available on bed, engage mechanism to make the bed surface firmer for repositioning.	
___	___	___	12. **Fold or bunch the drawsheet close to the patient before grasping it securely and preparing to move the patient.**	
___	___	___	13. Flex your knees and hips. Tighten your abdominal and gluteal muscles and keep your back straight.	

Moving a Patient Up in Bed With the Assistance of Another Nurse *(Continued)*

Excellent	Satisfactory	Needs Practice		Comments
___	___	___	14. **Shift your weight back and forth from your back leg to your front leg and count to three. On the count of three, move the patient up in bed. If possible, the patient can assist with the move by pushing with the legs.** Repeat the process if necessary to get the patient to the right position.	
___	___	___	15. Assist the patient to a comfortable position and readjust the pillows and supports as needed. Return bed surface to normal position, if necessary. Raise the side rails. Place the bed in the lowest position.	
___	___	___	16. Remove gloves if used and perform hand hygiene.	

Skill Checklists to Accompany Fundamentals of Nursing:
The Art and Science of Nursing Care, 6th edition

Name _____   Date _____

Unit _____   Position _____

Instructor/Evaluator: _____   Position _____

Excellent	Satisfactory	Needs Practice	SKILL 39-4 **Transferring a Patient From the Bed to a Stretcher**

SKILL 39-4

Transferring a Patient From the Bed to a Stretcher

Goal: The patient is transferred without injury to patient or nurse.   **Comments**

Excellent	Satisfactory	Needs Practice		Comments
――	――	――	1. Review the medical record and nursing plan of care for conditions that may influence the patient's ability to move or to be positioned. Assess for tubes, intravenous lines, incisions, or equipment that may alter the positioning procedure. Identify any movement limitations. Consult patient handling algorithm, if available, to plan appropriate approach to moving the patient.	
――	――	――	2. Identify the patient. Explain the procedure to the patient.	
――	――	――	3. Perform hand hygiene and put on gloves, if necessary.	
――	――	――	4. Close the room door or curtains. Adjust the head of the bed to a flat position or as low as the patient can tolerate. Raise the bed to a height 1/2 inch higher than the transport stretcher. Lower the side rails, if in place.	
――	――	――	5. Place the bath blanket over the patient and remove the top covers from underneath.	
――	――	――	6. If a friction-reducing sheet or drawsheet is not in place under the patient, place one under the patient's midsection. Have patient fold arms against chest and move chin to chest. Use the drawsheet to move the patient to the side of the bed where the stretcher will be placed.	
――	――	――	7. Position the stretcher next to and parallel to the bed. **Lock the wheels on the stretcher and the bed.**	
――	――	――	8. Remove the pillow from the bed and place it on the stretcher. The two nurses should stand on the stretcher side of the bed. The third nurse should stand on the side of the bed without the stretcher.	
――	――	――	9. Position the transfer board or other lateral-assist device under the patient. Use the drawsheet to roll the patient away from the stretcher. Slide the transfer board across the space between the stretcher and the bed, partially under the patient. Roll the patient onto his back, so he is partially on the transfer board.	

SKILL 39-4

Transferring a Patient From the Bed to a Stretcher *(Continued)*

Excellent	Satisfactory	Needs Practice		Comments
____	____	____	10. The nurse on the side of the bed without the stretcher should kneel on the bed, with his or her knee at the upper torso closer to the patient than the other knee. Fold or bunch the drawsheet close to the patient before grasping it securely in preparation for the transfer.	
____	____	____	11. Have one of the nurses on the stretcher side of the bed reach across the stretcher and grasp the drawsheet at the head and chest areas of the patient. If the transfer device used has long handles, each nurse should grasp two of the handles.	
____	____	____	12. Have the other nurse reach across the stretcher and grasp the drawsheet at the patient's waist and thigh area.	
____	____	____	13. **At a signal given by one of the nurses, have the nurses standing on the stretcher side of the bed pull the sheet. At the same time, the nurse (or nurses) kneeling on the bed should lift the drawsheet, transferring the patient's weight toward the transfer board, and pushing the patient from the bed to the stretcher.**	
____	____	____	14. Once the patient is transferred to the stretcher, remove the transfer board, and secure the patient until the side rails are raised. Raise the side rails. Ensure the patient's comfort. Cover the patient with a blanket and remove the bath blanket from underneath. Leave the friction-reducing sheet or drawsheet in place for the return transfer.	
____	____	____	15. Remove gloves (if used) and perform hand hygiene.	

Skill Checklists to Accompany Fundamentals of Nursing:
The Art and Science of Nursing Care, 6th edition

Name _____ Date _____

Unit _____ Position _____

Instructor/Evaluator: _____ Position _____

SKILL 39-5

Transferring a Patient From the Bed to a Chair

Goal: The transfer is accomplished without injury to patient or nurse and the patient remains free of any complications of immobility.

Excellent	Satisfactory	Needs Practice		Comments
___	___	___	1. Review the medical record and nursing plan of care for conditions that may influence the patient's ability to move or to be positioned. Assess for tubes, intravenous lines, incisions, or equipment that may alter the positioning procedure. Identify any movement limitations. Consult patient handling algorithm, if available, to plan appropriate approach to moving the patient.	
___	___	___	2. Identify the patient. Explain the procedure to the patient.	
___	___	___	3. Perform hand hygiene and put on gloves, if necessary.	
___	___	___	4. If needed, move equipment to make room for the chair. Close the door or draw the curtains.	
___	___	___	5. Place the bed in the lowest position. Raise the head of the bed to a sitting position or as high as the patient can tolerate.	
___	___	___	6. **Make sure the bed brakes are locked. Put the chair next to the bed, facing the foot of the bed. If available, lock the brakes of the chair. If the chair does not have brakes, brace the chair against a secure object.**	
___	___	___	7. Encourage the patient to make use of a stand-assist aid, either free-standing or attached to the side of the bed, if available, to move to the side of the bed and to a side-lying position, facing the side of the bed the patient will sit on.	
___	___	___	8. Lower the side rail if necessary and stand near the patient's hips. Stand with your legs shoulder width apart with one foot near the head of the bed, slightly in front of the other foot.	
___	___	___	9. Encourage the patient to make use of the stand-assist device. Assist the patient to sit up on the side of the bed; ask the patient to swing his or her legs over the side of the bed. At the same time, pivot on your back leg to lift the patient's trunk and shoulders. **Keep your back straight; avoid twisting.**	

Excellent	Satisfactory	Needs Practice		SKILL 39-5 **Transferring a Patient From the Bed to a Chair** (*Continued*)	
					Comments
___	___	___	10.	Stand in front of the patient and assess for any balance problems or complaints of dizziness. Allow legs to dangle a few minutes before continuing.	
___	___	___	11.	Assist the patient to put on a robe and nonskid footwear.	
___	___	___	12.	Wrap the gait belt around the patient's waist, based on assessed need and facility policy.	
___	___	___	13.	Stand facing the patient. Spread your feet about shoulder width apart and flex your hips and knees.	
___	___	___	14.	Ask the patient to slide his or her buttocks to the edge of the bed until the feet touch the floor. Position yourself as close as possible to the patient, with your foot positioned on the outside of the patient's foot. If a second staff person is assisting, have him/her assume a similar position.	
___	___	___	15.	Encourage the patient to make use of the stand-assist device. If necessary, have second staff person grasp the gait belt on the opposite side. Using the gait belt, assist the patient to stand. Rock back and forth while counting to three. **On the count of three, use your legs (not your back) to help raise the patient to a standing position. If indicated, brace your front knee against the patient's weak extremity as he or she stands.** Assess the patient's balance and leg strength. If the patient is weak or unsteady, return the patient to bed.	
___	___	___	16.	Pivot on your back foot and assist the patient to turn until the patient feels the chair against his or her legs.	
___	___	___	17.	Ask the patient to use an arm to steady himself or herself on the arm of the chair while slowly lowering to a sitting position. Continue to brace the patient's knees with your knees and hold the gait belt. Flex your hips and knees when helping the patient sit in the chair.	
___	___	___	18.	Assess the patient's alignment in the chair. Remove gait belt, if desired. Depending on patient comfort, it could be left in place to use when returning to bed. Cover with a blanket if needed. Place the call bell close.	
___	___	___	19.	Remove gloves if used and perform hand hygiene.	

Skill Checklists to Accompany Fundamentals of Nursing:
The Art and Science of Nursing Care, 6th edition

Name _____   Date _____

Unit _____   Position _____

Instructor/Evaluator: _____   Position _____

SKILL 41-1
Giving a Back Massage

Goal: The patient reports increased comfort and/or decreased pain and the patient is relaxed.

Excellent	Satisfactory	Needs Practice		Comments
——	——	——	1. Identify the patient. Offer a back massage to the patient and explain the procedure.	
——	——	——	2. Perform hand hygiene and put on nonsterile gloves, if indicated.	
——	——	——	3. Close room door and/or curtain.	
——	——	——	4. Assess the patient's pain, using an appropriate assessment tool and measurement scale.	
——	——	——	5. Raise the bed to a comfortable working height and lower the side rail nearest you.	
——	——	——	6. Assist the patient to a comfortable position, preferably the prone or side-lying position. Remove the covers and move the patient's gown just enough to expose the patient's back from the shoulders to sacral area. Drape the patient as needed with the bath blanket.	
——	——	——	7. **Warm the lubricant or lotion in the palm of your hand, or place the container in small basin of warm water.**	
——	——	——	8. Using light gliding strokes (*effleurage*), apply lotion to patient's shoulders, back, and sacral area.	
——	——	——	9. Place your hands beside each other at the base of the patient's spine and stroke upward to the shoulders and back downward to the buttocks in slow, continuous strokes. Continue for several minutes.	
——	——	——	10. Massage the patient's shoulder, entire back, areas over iliac crests, and sacrum with circular stroking motions. **Keep your hands in contact with the patient's skin.** Continue for several minutes, applying additional lotion as necessary.	
——	——	——	11. Knead the patient's skin by gently alternating grasping and compression motions (*pétrissage*).	
——	——	——	12. Complete the massage with additional long stroking movements that eventually become lighter in pressure.	
——	——	——	13. During massage, observe the patient's skin for reddened or open areas. **Pay particular attention to the skin over bony prominences.**	

Giving a Back Massage *(Continued)*

Excellent	Satisfactory	Needs Practice		Comments
___	___	___	14. Use the towel to pat the patient dry and to remove excess lotion. Apply powder if the patient requests it.	
___	___	___	15. Reposition patient gown and covers. Raise side rail and lower bed. Assist patient to a position of comfort.	
___	___	___	16. Remove gloves, if worn, and perform hand hygiene.	
___	___	___	17. Evaluate the patient's response to interventions. Reassess level of discomfort or pain using original assessment tools. Reassess and alter plan of care as appropriate.	

98

*Skill Checklists to Accompany Fundamentals of Nursing:
The Art and Science of Nursing Care, 6th edition*

Name _____   Date _____

Unit _____   Position _____

Instructor/Evaluator: _____   Position _____

Excellent	Satisfactory	Needs Practice	SKILL 42-1 **Inserting a Nasogastric Tube**	
			Goal: The tube is passed into the patient's stomach without any complications.	**Comments**
——	——	——	1. Check physician's order for insertion of NG tube and consider the risks associated with nasogastric tube insertion.	
——	——	——	2. Identify the patient.	
——	——	——	3. Explain the procedure to the patient and provide rationale as to why the tube is needed. Discuss the associated discomforts that may be experienced and possible interventions that may ally this discomfort. Answer any questions as needed.	
——	——	——	4. Gather equipment including selection of the appropriate NG polyurethane tube.	
——	——	——	5. Perform hand hygiene. Put on nonsterile gloves.	
——	——	——	6. Close the patient's bedside curtain or door. Raise the bed. Assist the patient to high Fowler's position and elevate the head of the bed 45 degrees. Drape chest with bath towel or disposable pad. Have emesis basin and tissues handy.	
——	——	——	7. **Measure the distance to insert tube by placing tip of tube at patient's nostril and extending to tip of ear lobe and then to tip of xiphoid process.** Mark tube with an indelible marker.	
——	——	——	8. Lubricate tip of tube (at least 2″ to 4″) with water-soluble lubricant. Apply topical anesthetic to nostril and oropharynx, as appropriate.	
——	——	——	9. After selecting the appropriate nostril, ask the patient to slightly flex head back against the pillow. Gently insert the tube into the nostril while directing the tube upward and backward along the floor of the nose. The patient may gag when the tube reaches the pharynx. Provide tissues for tearing or watering of eyes. Offer comfort and reassurance to the patient.	

Copyright © 2008 by Lippincott Williams & Wilkins. *Skill Checklists to Accompany Fundamentals of Nursing: The Art and Science of Nursing Care*, 6th edition, by Carol Taylor, Carol Lillis, Priscilla LeMone, Pamela Lynn, and Marilee LeBon.

SKILL 42-1
Inserting a Nasogastric Tube *(Continued)*

Excellent	Satisfactory	Needs Practice		Comments
——	——	——	10. **When pharynx is reached, instruct the patient to touch chin to chest.** Encourage the patient to sip water through a straw or swallow, even if no fluids are permitted. Advance the tube in a downward and backward direction when the patient swallows. Stop when the patient breathes. **If gagging and coughing persist, stop advancing the tube and check placement of tube with tongue blade and flashlight.** If the tube is curled, straighten the tube and attempt to advance again. Keep advancing the tube until pen marking is reached. **Do not use force. Rotate the tube if it meets resistance.**	
——	——	——	11. **Discontinue procedure and remove tube if there are signs of distress, such as gasping, coughing, cyanosis, and inability to speak or hum.**	
——	——	——	12. **While keeping one hand on the tube or temporarily securing with tape, determine that the tube is in patient's stomach:**	
——	——	——	a. Attach syringe to end of tube and aspirate a small amount of fluid.	
——	——	——	b. Measure the pH of aspirated fluid using pH paper or a meter. Place a drop of gastric secretions onto pH paper or place small amount in plastic cup and dip the pH paper into it. Within 30 seconds, compare the color on the paper with the chart supplied by the manufacturer.	
——	——	——	c. Visualize aspirated contents, checking for color and consistency.	
——	——	——	d. Obtain radiograph (x-ray) of placement of tube (as ordered by physician).	
——	——	——	13. Apply tincture of benzoin or other skin adhesive to tip of nose and allow to dry. Secure tube with tape to patient's nose:	
——	——	——	a. Cut a 4″ piece of tape and split bottom 2″ or use packaged nose tape for NG tubes.	
——	——	——	b. Place unsplit end over bridge of patient's nose.	
——	——	——	c. Wrap split ends under tubing and up and over onto nose. **Be careful not to pull tube too tightly against nose.**	
——	——	——	14. Clamp tube and cap or attach tube to suction according to the physician's orders.	

Inserting a Nasogastric Tube *(Continued)*

Excellent	Satisfactory	Needs Practice		Comments
—	—	—	15. Secure tube to patient's gown by using rubber band or tape and safety pin. For additional support, tube can be taped onto patient's cheek using a piece of tape. **If double-lumen tube (eg, Salem sump) is used, secure vent above stomach level. Attach at shoulder level.**	
—	—	—	16. Assist with or provide oral hygiene at 2- to 4-hour intervals. Lubricate the lips generously and clean nares and lubricate as needed. Offer analgesic throat lozenges or anesthetic spray for throat irritation if needed.	
—	—	—	17. Remove all equipment, lower the bed, and make the patient comfortable. Remove nonsterile gloves and perform hand hygiene.	

Skill Checklists to Accompany Fundamentals of Nursing:
The Art and Science of Nursing Care, 6th edition

Name _____   Date _____

Unit _____   Position _____

Instructor/Evaluator: _____   Position _____

Excellent	Satisfactory	Needs Practice	SKILL 42-2 **Administering a Tube Feeding**	Comments
			Goal: The patient will receive the tube feeding without complaints of nausea, or episodes of vomiting.	
___	___	___	1. Identify the patient.	
___	___	___	2. Explain the procedure to the patient and why this intervention is needed. Raise the bed. Pull the patient's bedside curtain. Perform key abdominal assessments as described above.	
___	___	___	3. Assemble equipment. Check amount, concentration, type, and frequency of tube feeding on patient's chart. Check expiration date of formula.	
___	___	___	4. Perform hand hygiene. Put on nonsterile gloves.	
___	___	___	5. **Position the patient with the head of the bed elevated at least 30 to 45 degrees or as near normal position for eating as possible.**	
___	___	___	6. Unpin tube from the patient's gown. **Check to see that the NG tube is properly located in the stomach, by first instilling air, then aspirate for gastric contents.** At times, due to the tendency of small bore tubes to collapse upon aspiration, several attempts may be necessary to aspirate gastric contents. After repeated instillations of 30 mL of air, accompanied by repositioning the patient, if you are unable to aspirate gastric contents, the tube placement should be checked by radiograph verified by physician's order. Check the pH as described in Guidelines for Nursing Care 42-1.	
___	___	___	7. After multiple steps have been taken to ensure that the feeding tube is located in the stomach or small intestine, **aspirate all gastric contents with a syringe and measure to check for the residual amount of feeding in the stomach.** Flush tube with 30 mL of water for irrigation. Proceed with feeding if amount of residual does not exceed agency policy or physician's guideline. Disconnect syringe from tubing and cap end of tubing while preparing the formula feeding equipment. Remove gloves.	
___	___	___	8. Put on nonsterile gloves before preparing, assembling, and handling any part of the feeding system.	
___	___	___	9. Administer feeding.	

SKILL 42-2
Administering a Tube Feeding *(Continued)*

Excellent	Satisfactory	Needs Practice		Comments

When Using a Feeding Bag (Open System)

——— ——— ———   a. Hang bag on IV pole and adjust to about 12″ above the stomach. Clamp tubing.

——— ——— ———   b. Check the expiration date of the formula. Cleanse top of feeding container with a disinfectant before opening it. **Pour formula into feeding bag and allow solution to run through tubing.** Close clamp.

——— ——— ———   c. Attach feeding setup to feeding tube, open clamp, and regulate drip according to physician's order, or allow feeding to run in over 30 minutes.

——— ——— ———   d. **Add 30 to 60 mL (1 to 2 oz) of water for irrigation to feeding bag when feeding is almost completed and allow it to run through the tube.**

——— ——— ———   e. Clamp tubing immediately after water has been instilled. Disconnect from feeding tube. Clamp tube and cover end with cap.

When Using a Large Syringe (Open System)

——— ——— ———   a. Remove plunger from 30- or 60-mL syringe.

——— ——— ———   b. Attach syringe to feeding tube, pour premeasured amount of tube feeding into syringe, open clamp, and allow food to enter tube. **Regulate rate, fast or slow, by height of the syringe. Do not push formula with syringe plunger.**

——— ——— ———   c. **Add 30 to 60 mL (1 to 2 oz) of water for irrigation to syringe when feeding is almost completed and allow it to run through the tube.**

——— ——— ———   d. When syringe has emptied, hold syringe high and disconnect from tube. Clamp tube and cover end with cap.

When Using an Enteral Feeding Pump

——— ——— ———   a. Close flow-regulator clamp on tubing and fill feeding bag with prescribed formula. Amount used depends on agency policy. Place label on container with patient's name and date and time the feeding was hung.

——— ——— ———   b. Hang feeding container on IV pole. **Allow solution to flow through tubing.**

Excellent	Satisfactory	Needs Practice	SKILL 42-2 **Administering a Tube Feeding** *(Continued)*	
				Comments
—	—	—	c. Connect to feeding pump following manufacturer's directions. Set rate. Maintain the patient in the upright position throughout the feeding. If the patient needs to temporarily lie flat, the feeding should be paused. The feeding may be resumed after the patient's position has been changed back to 30 to 45 degrees.	
—	—	—	d. **Check residual every 4 to 8 hours.**	
—	—	—	10. Observe the patient's response during and after tube feeding and assess the abdomen at least once a shift.	
—	—	—	11. **Have the patient remain in an upright position for at least 1 hour after feeding.**	
—	—	—	12. Wash and clean equipment or replace according to agency policy. Remove gloves and perform hand hygiene.	

Skill Checklists to Accompany Fundamentals of Nursing:
The Art and Science of Nursing Care, 6th edition

Name _____   Date _____

Unit _____   Position _____

Instructor/Evaluator: _____   Position _____

SKILL 42-3
Removing a Nasogastric Tube

Goal: The tube is removed with minimal discomfort to the patient, and the patient maintains an adequate nutritional intake.

Excellent	Satisfactory	Needs Practice		Comments
___	___	___	1. Check physician's order for removal of NG tube.	
___	___	___	2. Identify the patient.	
___	___	___	3. Explain the procedure to the patient and why this intervention is warranted. Describe that it will entail a quick few moments of discomfort. Perform key abdominal assessments as described above.	
___	___	___	4. Gather equipment.	
___	___	___	5. Perform hand hygiene. Put on nonsterile disposable gloves.	
___	___	___	6. Pull the patient's bedside curtain. Raise the bed to the appropriate height and place the patient in a 30- to 45-degree position. Place a towel or disposable pad across the patient's chest. Give tissues and emesis basin to the patient.	
___	___	___	7. Discontinue suction and separate tube from suction. Unpin tube from the patient's gown and carefully remove adhesive tape from the patient's nose.	
___	___	___	8. Check placement and **attach syringe and flush with 10 mL of water or normal saline solution (optional) or clear with 30 to 50 mL of air.**	
___	___	___	9. Instruct the patient to take a deep breath and hold it.	
___	___	___	10. **Clamp tube with fingers by doubling tube on itself. Quickly and carefully remove tube while the patient holds breath. Coil the tube in a disposable towel as you remove it from the patient.**	
___	___	___	11. Dispose of tube per agency policy. Remove gloves and place in bag. Perform hand hygiene.	
___	___	___	12. Offer mouth care to patient and facial tissue to blow nose. Lower the bed and assist the patient to a position of comfort as needed.	

Excellent	Satisfactory	Needs Practice	SKILL 42-3 **Removing a Nasogastric Tube** *(Continued)*	
				Comments
——	——	——	13. Put on gloves and measure the amount of nasogastric drainage in the collection device and record on output flow record, subtracting irrigant fluids if necessary. Add solidifying agent to nasogastric drainage according to hospital policy.	
——	——	——	14. Remove gloves and perform hand hygiene.	

Skill Checklists to Accompany *Fundamentals of Nursing:
The Art and Science of Nursing Care*, 6th edition

Name _____ Date _____

Unit _____ Position _____

Instructor/Evaluator: _____ Position _____

SKILL 42-4
Irrigating a Nasogastric Tube Connected to Suction

Goal: The tube will maintain patency with irrigation.

Excellent	Satisfactory	Needs Practice		Comments
—	—	—	1. Check the physician's order.	
—	—	—	2. Identify the patient.	
—	—	—	3. Explain the procedure to the patient and why this intervention is warranted. Perform key abdominal assessments as described above.	
—	—	—	4. Gather necessary equipment. Check expiration dates on irrigating solution and irrigation set.	
—	—	—	5. Perform hand hygiene. Put on gloves.	
—	—	—	6. Pull the patient's bedside curtain. Raise the bed. Assist patient to a 30- to 45-degree position, unless this is contraindicated.	
—	—	—	7. **Check placement of NG tube.** (Refer to Skill 42-1.)	
—	—	—	8. Pour irrigating solution into container. Draw up 30 mL of saline solution (or the amount ordered by physician) into syringe.	
—	—	—	9. Clamp suction tubing near connection site. If needed, disconnect tube from suction apparatus and lay on disposable pad or towel, or hold both tubes upright in nondominant hand.	
—	—	—	10. Place tip of syringe in tube. **If Salem sump or double-lumen tube is used, make sure that syringe tip is placed in drainage port and not in blue air vent.** Hold syringe upright and gently insert the irrigant (or allow solution to flow in by gravity if agency policy or physician indicates). **Do not force solution into tube.**	
—	—	—	11. **If unable to irrigate tube, reposition the patient and attempt irrigation again. Inject 10 to 20 mL of air and aspirate again. Check with physician or follow agency policy if repeated attempts to irrigate tube fail.**	

Excellent	Satisfactory	Needs Practice		Comments
——	——	——	12. After irrigant has been instilled, observe for return flow of NG drainage into available container. Alternately, the nurse may reconnect the NG tube to suction and observe the return drainage as it drains into the suction container. **Inject air into blue air vent after irrigation is complete. Position the blue air vent above the patient's stomach.**	
——	——	——	13. Measure and record amount and description of irrigant and returned solution if measured at this time.	
——	——	——	14. Rinse equipment if it will be reused. Label with the date, patient's name, room number, and purpose (for NG tube/irrigation). Remove gloves and perform hand hygiene.	
——	——	——	15. Lower the bed. Assist the patient to a position of comfort. Perform hand hygiene.	

Skill Checklists to Accompany Fundamentals of Nursing:
The Art and Science of Nursing Care, 6th edition

Name _____   Date _____

Unit _____   Position _____

Instructor/Evaluator: _____   Position _____

Excellent	Satisfactory	Needs Practice	SKILL 42-5 **Obtaining a Capillary Blood Sample for Glucose Testing**	
			Goal: Patient blood glucose levels are accurately monitored.	**Comments**
——	——	——	1. Check the patient's medical record or nursing care plan for monitoring schedule. You may decide that additional testing is indicated based on nursing judgment and the patient's condition.	
——	——	——	2. Gather equipment.	
——	——	——	3. Close curtains around bed and close door to room if possible.	
——	——	——	4. Identify the patient. Explain procedure to the patient and instruct the patient about the need for monitoring blood glucose.	
——	——	——	5. Perform hand hygiene. Put on nonsterile gloves.	
——	——	——	6. Turn on the monitor.	
——	——	——	7. Enter the patient's identification number, if required, according to facility policy.	
——	——	——	8. Prepare lancet using aseptic technique.	
——	——	——	9. Remove test strip from the vial. **Recap container immediately.** Test strips also come individually wrapped. Turn on monitor. **Check that code number for the strip matches code number on monitor screen.**	
——	——	——	10. Insert strip into the meter according to directions for that specific device.	
——	——	——	11. For adult, massage side of finger toward puncture site.	
——	——	——	12. **Have the patient wash hands with soap and warm water and dry thoroughly. Alternately, the skin may be cleansed with an alcohol swab. Allow skin to dry completely.**	
——	——	——	13. Hold lancet perpendicular to skin and prick site with lancet.	
——	——	——	14. **Wipe away first drop of blood with gauze square or cotton ball if recommended by manufacturer of monitor.**	

SKILL 42-5

Obtaining a Capillary Blood Sample for
Glucose Testing *(Continued)*

Excellent	Satisfactory	Needs Practice		Comments
——	——	——	15. Encourage bleeding by lowering hand, making use of gravity. Lightly stroke the finger, if necessary, until a sufficient amount of blood has formed to cover the sample area on the strip, based on monitor requirements (check instructions for monitor). Take care not to squeeze the finger, squeeze at puncture site, or to touch puncture site or blood.	
——	——	——	16. **Gently touch drop of blood to pad on test strip without smearing it.**	
——	——	——	17. Press time button if directed by manufacturer.	
——	——	——	18. Apply pressure to puncture site with a cotton ball. **Do not use alcohol wipe.**	
——	——	——	19. Read blood glucose results and document appropriately at bedside. Inform patient of test result.	
——	——	——	20. Turn meter off, remove test strip, and dispose of supplies appropriately. Place lancet in sharps container.	
——	——	——	21. Remove gloves and perform hand hygiene.	

Skill Checklists to Accompany Fundamentals of Nursing:
The Art and Science of Nursing Care, 6th edition

Name _____   Date _____

Unit _____   Position _____

Instructor/Evaluator: _____   Position _____

Excellent	Satisfactory	Needs Practice	SKILL 43-1 **Assisting With the Use of a Bedpan** **Goal:** The patient is able to void with assistance.	Comments
____	____	____	1. Identify the patient. Discuss procedure with the patient and assess the patient's ability to assist with the procedure, as well as personal hygiene preferences. Review chart for any limitations in physical activity.	
____	____	____	2. Bring bedpan and other necessary equipment to bedside. Perform hand hygiene. Put on disposable gloves.	
____	____	____	3. Warm bedpan, if it is made of metal, by rinsing it with warm water.	
____	____	____	4. Unless contraindicated, apply powder to the rim of the bedpan.	
____	____	____	5. Place bedpan and cover on chair next to bed. Close curtains around bed and close door to room if possible.	
____	____	____	6. If bed is adjustable, place it in high position. Place the patient in a supine position, with the head of the bed elevated about 30 degrees, unless contraindicated.	
____	____	____	7. Fold top linen back just enough to allow placement of bedpan. If there is no waterproof pad on the bed and time allows, consider placing a waterproof pad under the patient's buttocks before placing bedpan.	
____	____	____	8. Ask the patient to bend the knees. Have the patient lift his or her hips upward. Assist the patient, if necessary, by placing your hand that is closest to the patient palm up, under the lower back and assist with lifting. Slip the bedpan into place with other hand.	
____	____	____	9. **Ensure that bedpan is in proper position and the patient's buttocks are resting on the rounded shelf of the regular bedpan or the shallow rim of the fracture bedpan.**	
____	____	____	10. Raise head of bed as near to sitting position as tolerated, unless contraindicated. Cover the patient with bed linens.	
____	____	____	11. **Place call device and toilet tissue within easy reach. Place the bed in the lowest position.** Leave the patient if it is safe to do so. Use side rails appropriately.	
____	____	____	12. Remove gloves and perform hand hygiene.	

Excellent	Satisfactory	Needs Practice	SKILL 43-1 **Assisting With the Use of a Bedpan** *(Continued)*	Comments
			Removing the Bedpan	
――	――	――	13. Perform hand hygiene and put on disposable gloves. Raise the bed to a comfortable working height. Have a receptacle, such as plastic trash bag, handy for discarding tissue.	
――	――	――	14. Lower the head of the bed, if necessary, to about 30 degrees. Remove bedpan in the same manner in which it was offered, being careful to hold it steady. Ask the patient to bend the knees and lift the buttocks up from the bedpan. Assist the patient, if necessary, by placing your hand that is closest to the patient palm up, under the lower back and assist with lifting. Place the bedpan on the bedside chair and cover it.	
――	――	――	15. If the patient needs assistance with hygiene, wrap tissue around the hand several times, and wipe the patient clean, using one stroke from the pubic area toward the anal area. Discard tissue, and use more until the patient is clean. Place the patient on his or her side and spread buttocks to clean the anal area.	
――	――	――	16. Do not place toilet tissue in the bedpan if a specimen is required or if output is being recorded. Place toilet tissue in appropriate receptacle.	
――	――	――	17. Return the patient to a comfortable position. Make sure the linens under the patient are dry. Replace or remove pad under the patient as necessary. Remove your gloves and ensure that the patient is covered.	
――	――	――	18. Raise side rail. Lower bed height and adjust head of bed to a comfortable position. Reattach call bell.	
――	――	――	19. Offer the patient supplies to wash and dry his or her hands, assisting as necessary.	
――	――	――	20. Put on clean gloves. Empty and clean the bedpan, measuring urine in graduated container, as necessary. Discard trash receptacle with used toilet paper per facility policy. Perform hand hygiene.	

Skill Checklists to Accompany Fundamentals of Nursing:
The Art and Science of Nursing Care, 6th edition

Name _____ Date _____

Unit _____ Position _____

Instructor/Evaluator: _____ Position _____

SKILL 43-2
Assisting With the Use of a Urinal

Excellent	Satisfactory	Needs Practice	**Goal:** The patient is able to void with assistance.	Comments
—	—	—	1. Identify the patient. Discuss procedure with the patient and assess the patient's ability to assist with the procedure, as well as personal hygiene preferences. Review chart for any limitations in physical activity.	
—	—	—	2. Bring urinal and other necessary equipment to bedside. Perform hand hygiene. Put on disposable gloves.	
—	—	—	3. Close curtains around bed and close door to room if possible.	
—	—	—	4. Assist the patient to an appropriate position as necessary: standing at the bedside, lying on one side or his back, sitting in bed with the head elevated, or sitting on the side of the bed.	
—	—	—	5. If the patient remains in the bed, fold the linens just enough to allow for proper placement of the urinal.	
—	—	—	6. If the patient is not standing, have him spread his legs slightly. **Hold the urinal close to the penis and position the penis completely within the urinal. Keep the bottom of the urinal lower than the penis. If necessary, assist the patient to hold the urinal in place.**	
—	—	—	7. Cover the patient with the bed linens.	
—	—	—	8. Place call device and toilet tissue within easy reach. Have a receptacle, such as plastic trash bag, handy for discarding tissue. Place the bed in the lowest position. Leave the patient if it is safe to do so. Use side rails appropriately.	
—	—	—	9. Remove gloves and perform hand hygiene.	
			Removing the Urinal	
—	—	—	10. Perform hand hygiene and put on disposable gloves.	
—	—	—	11. Pull back the patient's bed linens just enough to remove the urinal. Cover the open end of the urinal. Place on the bedside chair. If patient needs assistance with hygiene, wrap tissue around the hand several times, and wipe patient clean. Place tissue in receptacle.	

Excellent	Satisfactory	Needs Practice		Comments
			SKILL 43-2 **Assisting With the Use of a Urinal** *(Continued)*	
___	___	___	12. Return the patient to a comfortable position. Make sure the linens under the patient are dry. Remove your gloves and ensure that the patient is covered.	
___	___	___	13. Ensure the patient call bell is within reach.	
___	___	___	14. Offer the patient supplies to wash and dry his hands, assisting as necessary.	
___	___	___	15. Put on clean gloves. Empty and clean the urinal, measuring urine in graduated container, as necessary. Discard trash receptacle with used toilet paper per facility policy. Remove gloves and perform hand hygiene.	

Skill Checklists to Accompany Fundamentals of Nursing:
The Art and Science of Nursing Care, 6th edition

Name _____ Date _____

Unit _____ Position _____

Instructor/Evaluator: _____ Position _____

Excellent	Satisfactory	Needs Practice	SKILL 43-3 **Assessing Bladder Volume Using an Ultrasound Bladder Scanner** **Goal:** The volume of urine in the bladder will be accurately measured.	Comments
——	——	——	1. Identify the patient. Discuss procedure with the patient. Review chart for any limitations in physical activity.	
——	——	——	2. Bring the bladder scanner and other necessary equipment to bedside. Obtain assistance from another staff member, if necessary. Perform hand hygiene.	
——	——	——	3. Close curtains around bed and close door to room if possible.	
——	——	——	4. Raise the bed to a comfortable working height. Stand on the patient's right side if you are right handed or the patient's left side if you are left handed.	
——	——	——	5. Assist the patient to a supine position. Drape the patient.	
——	——	——	6. Put on clean gloves.	
——	——	——	7. Press the "On" button. Wait until the device warms up. Press the "Scan" button to turn on the scanning screen.	
——	——	——	8. Press the appropriate gender button. The appropriate icon for male or female will appear on the screen.	
——	——	——	9. Clean the scanner head with the appropriate cleaner.	
——	——	——	10. **Gently palpate the patient's symphysis pubis. Place a generous amount of ultrasound gel or gel pad midline on the patient's abdomen, about 1″ to 1½″ above the symphysis pubis (anterior midline junction of pubic bones).**	
——	——	——	11. **Place the scanner head on the gel or gel pad, with the directional icon on the scanner head toward the patient's head. Aim the scanner head toward the bladder (point the scanner head slightly downward toward the coccyx). Press and release the "Scan" button.**	
——	——	——	12. Observe the image on the scanner screen. **Adjust the scanner head to center the bladder image on the crossbars.**	

Assessing Bladder Volume Using an Ultrasound Bladder Scanner *(Continued)*

Excellent	Satisfactory	Needs Practice		Comments
——	——	——	13. Press and hold the "Done" button until it beeps. Read the volume measurement on the screen. Print the results if required by pressing "Print."	
——	——	——	14. Use a washcloth or paper towel to remove remaining gel from the patient's skin. Alternately, gently remove gel pad from the patient's skin. Return the patient to a comfortable position. Remove your gloves and ensure that the patient is covered.	

Skill Checklists to Accompany Fundamentals of Nursing:
The Art and Science of Nursing Care, 6th edition

Name _____ Date _____

Unit _____ Position _____

Instructor/Evaluator: _____ Position _____

SKILL 43-4

Catheterizing the Female Urinary Bladder

Goal: The patient's urinary elimination will be maintained, with a urine output of at least 30 mL/hour, and the patient's bladder will not be distended.

Excellent	Satisfactory	Needs Practice		Comments
——	——	——	1. Identify the patient. Discuss procedure with the patient and assess the patient's ability to assist with the procedure. Discuss any allergies with patient, especially to iodine and latex. Review chart for any limitations in physical activity.	
——	——	——	2. Bring the catheter kit and other necessary equipment to bedside. Obtain assistance from another staff member, if necessary. Perform hand hygiene.	
——	——	——	3. Close curtains around bed and close door to room if possible.	
——	——	——	4. Provide for good light. Artificial light is recommended (use of a flashlight requires an assistant to hold and position it). Place a trash receptacle within easy reach.	
——	——	——	5. Raise the bed to a comfortable working height. Stand on the patient's right side if you are right handed or on the patient's left side if you are left handed.	
——	——	——	6. Assist patient to dorsal recumbent position with knees flexed, feet about 2 feet apart, with her legs abducted. Drape the patient. Alternately, the Sims', or lateral, position can be used. Place the patient's buttocks near the edge of the bed with her shoulders at the opposite edge and her knees drawn toward her chest. Allow the patient to lie on either side, depending on which position is easiest for the nurse and best for the patient's comfort. Slide waterproof pad under the patient.	
——	——	——	7. Put on clean gloves. Clean the perineal area with washcloth, skin cleanser, and warm water, using a different corner of the washcloth with each stroke. Wipe from above orifice downward toward sacrum (front to back). Rinse and dry. Remove gloves. Perform hand hygiene again.	
——	——	——	8. Prepare urine drainage setup if a separate urine collection system is to be used. Secure to bed frame according to manufacturer's directions.	
——	——	——	9. Open sterile catheterization tray on a clean overbed table using sterile technique.	

Excellent	Satisfactory	Needs Practice		Comments
			SKILL 43-4 **Catheterizing the Female Urinary Bladder** *(Continued)*	

Excellent	Satisfactory	Needs Practice		Comments
⎯	⎯	⎯	10. Put on sterile gloves. Grasp upper corners of drape and unfold drape without touching unsterile areas. Fold back a corner on each side to make a cuff over gloved hands. Ask the patient to lift her buttocks and slide sterile drape under her with gloves protected by cuff.	
⎯	⎯	⎯	11. Place a fenestrated sterile drape over the perineal area, exposing the labia.	
⎯	⎯	⎯	12. Place sterile tray on drape between patient's thighs.	
⎯	⎯	⎯	13. Open all the supplies. **Test the catheter balloon by removing protective cap on tip of syringe and attaching syringe prefilled with sterile water to injection port. Inject appropriate amount of fluid. If balloon inflates properly, withdraw fluid and leave syringe attached to port.**	
⎯	⎯	⎯	14. Fluff cotton balls in tray before pouring antiseptic solution over them. Alternately, open package of antiseptic swabs. Open specimen container if specimen is to be obtained.	
⎯	⎯	⎯	15. Lubricate 1″ to 2″ of catheter tip.	
⎯	⎯	⎯	16. With thumb and one finger of nondominant hand, spread labia and identify meatus. **Be prepared to maintain separation of labia with one hand until catheter is inserted and urine is flowing well and continuously.** If the patient is in the side-lying position, lift the upper buttock and labia to expose the urinary meatus.	
⎯	⎯	⎯	17. Use your dominant hand to pick up a cotton ball. **Clean one labial fold, top to bottom (from above the meatus down toward the rectum), then discard the cotton ball. Using a new cotton ball for each stroke, continue to clean the other labial fold, then directly over the meatus.**	
⎯	⎯	⎯	18. With your uncontaminated, dominant hand, place drainage end of catheter in receptacle. If the catheter is preattached to sterile tubing and drainage container (closed drainage system), position catheter and setup within easy reach on sterile field. Ensure that clamp on drainage bag is closed.	
⎯	⎯	⎯	19. **Using your dominant hand, hold the catheter 2″ to 3″ from the tip and insert slowly into the urethra. Advance the catheter until there is a return of urine (approximately 2″ to 3″ [4.8 to 7.2 cm]). Once urine drains, advance catheter another 2″ to 3″ (4.8 to 7.2 cm). Do not force catheter through urethra into bladder.** Ask the patient to breathe deeply, and rotate catheter gently if slight resistance is met as catheter reaches external sphincter.	

SKILL 43-4

Catheterizing the Female Urinary Bladder *(Continued)*

Excellent	Satisfactory	Needs Practice		Comments
——	——	——	20. Hold the catheter securely at the meatus with your nondominant hand. Use your dominant hand to inflate the catheter balloon. Inject entire volume supplied in prefilled syringe.	
——	——	——	21. Pull gently on catheter after balloon is inflated to feel resistance.	
——	——	——	22. Attach catheter to drainage system if not already preattached.	
——	——	——	23. Remove equipment and dispose of according to facility policy. Wash and dry the perineal area as needed.	
——	——	——	24. Remove gloves. **Secure catheter tubing to the patient's inner thigh with Velcro leg strap or tape.** Leave some slack in catheter for leg movement.	
——	——	——	25. Assist the patient to a comfortable position. Cover the patient with bed linens. Place the bed in the lowest position.	
——	——	——	26. Secure drainage bag below the level of the bladder. Check that drainage tubing is not kinked and that movement of side rails does not interfere with catheter or drainage bag.	
——	——	——	27. Put on clean gloves. Obtain urine specimen immediately, if needed, from drainage bag. Label specimen. Send urine specimen to the laboratory promptly or refrigerate it.	
——	——	——	28. Remove gloves. Perform hand hygiene.	

Skill Checklists to Accompany Fundamentals of Nursing:
The Art and Science of Nursing Care, 6th edition

Name _____ Date _____

Unit _____ Position _____

Instructor/Evaluator: _____ Position _____

Excellent	Satisfactory	Needs Practice	SKILL 43-5 **Catheterizing the Male Urinary Bladder** **Goal:** The patient's urinary elimination will be maintained, with a urine output of at least 30 mL/hour, and the patient's bladder will not be distended.	Comments
____	____	____	1. Identify the patient. Discuss procedure with the patient and assess the patient's ability to assist with the procedure. Discuss any allergies with the patient, especially to iodine and latex. Review chart for any limitations in physical activity.	
____	____	____	2. Bring the catheter kit and other necessary equipment to bedside. Obtain assistance from another staff member, if necessary. Perform hand hygiene. Put on disposable gloves.	
____	____	____	3. Close curtains around bed and close door to room if possible.	
____	____	____	4. Provide for good light. Artificial light is recommended. Place a trash receptacle within easy reach.	
____	____	____	5. Raise the bed to a comfortable working height. Stand on the patient's right side if you are right handed or the patient's left side if you are left handed.	
____	____	____	6. Position the patient on his back with thighs slightly apart. Drape the patient so that only the area around the penis is exposed. Slide waterproof pad under the patient.	
____	____	____	7. Put on clean gloves. Clean the genital area with washcloth, skin cleanser, and warm water. Clean the tip of the penis first, moving the washcloth in a circular motion from the meatus outward. Wash the shaft of the penis using downward strokes toward the pubic area. Rinse and dry. Remove gloves. Perform hand hygiene again.	
____	____	____	8. Prepare urine drainage setup if a separate urine collection system is to be used. Secure to bed frame according to manufacturer's directions.	
____	____	____	9. Open sterile catheterization tray on a clean overbed table using sterile technique.	
____	____	____	10. Put on sterile gloves. Open sterile drape and place on patient's thighs. Place fenestrated drape with opening over penis.	
____	____	____	11. Place catheter set on or next to patient's legs on sterile drape.	

Catheterizing the Male Urinary Bladder *(Continued)*

Excellent	Satisfactory	Needs Practice		Comments
——	——	——	12. Open all the supplies. **Test the catheter balloon by removing protective cap on tip of syringe and attaching syringe prefilled with sterile water to injection port. Inject appropriate amount of fluid. If balloon inflates properly, withdraw fluid and leave syringe attached to port.**	
——	——	——	13. Fluff cotton balls in tray before pouring antiseptic solution over them. Alternately, open package of antiseptic swabs. Open specimen container if specimen is to be obtained.	
——	——	——	14. With your uncontaminated, dominant hand, place drainage end of catheter in receptacle. If the catheter is preattached to sterile tubing and drainage container (closed drainage system), position catheter and setup within easy reach on sterile field. Ensure that clamp on drainage bag is closed.	
——	——	——	15. Remove cap from syringe prefilled with lubricant.	
——	——	——	16. Lift penis with nondominant hand. Retract foreskin in uncircumcised patient. **Be prepared to keep this hand in this position until catheter is inserted and urine is flowing well and continuously. Using your dominant hand and the forceps, pick up a cotton ball. Using a circular motion, clean the penis, moving from the meatus down the glans of the penis. Repeat this cleansing motion two more times, using a new cotton ball each time. Discard each cotton ball after one use.**	
——	——	——	17. Hold the penis with slight upward tension and perpendicular to the patient's body. Use your dominant hand to pick up the lubricant syringe. **Gently insert tip of syringe with lubricant into urethra and instill the 10 mL of lubricant.**	
——	——	——	18. Use your dominant hand to pick up the catheter and hold it an inch or two from the tip. Ask the patient to bear down as if voiding. **Insert catheter tip into meatus. Ask the patient to take deep breaths as you advance the catheter to the bifurcation or Y level of the ports. Do not use force to introduce catheter.** If catheter resists entry, ask the patient to breathe deeply and rotate catheter slightly.	
——	——	——	19. Hold the catheter securely at the meatus with your nondominant hand. Use your dominant hand to inflate the catheter balloon. **Inject entire volume supplied in prefilled syringe. Once balloon is inflated, catheter may be gently pulled back into place. Replace foreskin over catheter.** Lower penis.	

SKILL 43-5
Catheterizing the Male Urinary Bladder *(Continued)*

Excellent	Satisfactory	Needs Practice		Comments
___	___	___	20. Pull gently on catheter after balloon is inflated to feel resistance.	
___	___	___	21. Attach catheter to drainage system if necessary.	
___	___	___	22. Remove equipment and dispose of according to facility policy. Wash and dry the perineal area as needed.	
___	___	___	23. Remove gloves. Secure catheter tubing to the patient's inner thigh or lower abdomen (with the penis directed toward the patient's chest) with Velcro leg strap or tape. Leave some slack in catheter for leg movement.	
___	___	___	24. Assist the patient to a comfortable position. Cover the patient with bed linens. Place the bed in the lowest position.	
___	___	___	25. Secure drainage bag below the level of the bladder. Check that drainage tubing is not kinked and that movement of side rails does not interfere with catheter or drainage bag.	
___	___	___	26. Put on clean gloves. Obtain urine specimen immediately, if needed, from drainage bag. Cover and label specimen. Send urine specimen to the laboratory promptly or refrigerate it.	
___	___	___	27. Remove gloves. Perform hand hygiene.	

Skill Checklists to Accompany Fundamentals of Nursing:
The Art and Science of Nursing Care, 6th edition

Name _____   Date _____

Unit _____   Position _____

Instructor/Evaluator: _____   Position _____

Excellent	Satisfactory	Needs Practice	SKILL 43-6 **Performing Intermittent Closed Catheter Irrigation** **Goal:** The patient exhibits the free flow of urine through the catheter.	Comments
——	——	——	1. Identify the patient. Discuss procedure with the patient.	
——	——	——	2. Perform hand hygiene.	
——	——	——	3. Provide privacy by closing the curtains or door and draping the patient with bath blanket.	
——	——	——	4. Raise the bed to a comfortable working height.	
——	——	——	5. Empty the catheter drainage bag and measure the amount of urine, noting the amount and characteristics of the urine.	
——	——	——	6. Assist the patient to comfortable position and expose access port on catheter setup. Place waterproof pad under catheter and aspiration port. Remove tape anchoring catheter to the patient.	
——	——	——	7. Open supplies, using aseptic technique. Pour sterile solution into sterile basin. Aspirate the prescribed amount of irrigant (usually 30 to 60 mL) into sterile syringe and attach capped, sterile, blunt-ended needle, if necessary. Put on gloves.	
——	——	——	8. **Cleanse the access port with antimicrobial swab.**	
——	——	——	9. Clamp or fold catheter tubing below the access port.	
——	——	——	10. Remove cap and insert needle into port. Alternately, attach the syringe to the port using a twisting motion, if needleless system is in place. **Gently instill solution into catheter.**	
——	——	——	11. Remove syringe/needle from port. Apply needle guard, if needle is used. **Unclamp or unfold tubing and allow irrigant and urine to flow into the drainage bag.** Repeat procedure as necessary.	
——	——	——	12. Remove gloves. Secure catheter tubing to the patient's inner thigh or lower abdomen (if a male patient) with Velcro leg strap or tape. Leave some slack in catheter for leg movement.	
——	——	——	13. Assist the patient to a comfortable position. Cover the patient with bed linens. Place the bed in the lowest position.	

SKILL 43-6
Performing Intermittent Closed Catheter Irrigation *(Continued)*

Excellent	Satisfactory	Needs Practice		Comments
—	—	—	14. Secure drainage bag below the level of the bladder. Check that drainage tubing is not kinked and that movement of side rails does not interfere with catheter or drainage bag.	
—	—	—	15. Remove equipment and discard needle and syringe in appropriate receptacle. Perform hand hygiene.	
—	—	—	16. Assess the patient's response to procedure and quality and amount of drainage after the irrigation.	

Skill Checklists to Accompany Fundamentals of Nursing:
The Art and Science of Nursing Care, 6th edition

Name _____   Date _____

Unit _____   Position _____

Instructor/Evaluator: _____   Position _____

Excellent	Satisfactory	Needs Practice	SKILL 43-7 **Administering a Continuous Closed Bladder Irrigation**	
			Goal: The patient exhibits free-flowing urine through the catheter.	**Comments**
——	——	——	1. Assemble equipment and double-check physician's order. Identify the patient. Discuss procedure with the patient.	
——	——	——	2. Calculate drip rate for prescribed infusion rate.	
——	——	——	3. Perform hand hygiene.	
——	——	——	4. Provide privacy by closing the curtains or door and draping the patient with bath blanket.	
——	——	——	5. Raise the bed to a comfortable working height.	
——	——	——	6. Empty the catheter drainage bag and measure the amount of urine, noting the amount and characteristics of the urine.	
——	——	——	7. Assist the patient to comfortable position and expose the irrigation port on the catheter setup. Place waterproof pad under catheter and aspiration port. Remove tape anchoring catheter to the patient.	
——	——	——	8. Prepare sterile irrigation bag for use as directed by manufacturer. Clearly label the solution as "Bladder Irrigant." Include the date and time on the label. Secure tubing clamp and attach sterile tubing with drip chamber to container using aseptic technique. Hang bag on IV pole 2.5 to 3 feet above level of the patient's bladder. Release clamp and remove protective cover on end of tubing without contaminating it. Allow solution to flush tubing and remove air. Clamp tubing and replace end cover.	
——	——	——	9. Put on gloves. **Cleanse the irrigation port with an alcohol swab. Using aseptic technique, attach irrigation tubing to irrigation port of three-way indwelling catheter.**	
——	——	——	10. Check the drainage tubing to make sure clamp, if present, is open.	
——	——	——	11. **Release clamp on irrigation tubing and regulate flow at determined drip rate, according to the physician's order.** At times, the physician may order the bladder irrigation to be done with a medicated solution. In these cases, use an IV pump to regulate the flow.	

SKILL 43-7

Administering a Continuous Closed
Bladder Irrigation *(Continued)*

Excellent	Satisfactory	Needs Practice		Comments
——	——	——	12. Remove gloves. Assist the patient to a comfortable position. Cover the patient with bed linens. Place the bed in the lowest position.	
——	——	——	13. Perform hand hygiene.	
——	——	——	14. Assess the patient's response to procedure and quality and amount of drainage.	
——	——	——	15. As irrigation fluid container nears empty, clamp the administration tubing. Do not allow drip chamber to empty. Disconnect empty bag and attach a new full irrigation solution bag. Continue as ordered by the physician.	
——	——	——	16. Record amount of irrigant used on intake/output record. Put on gloves and empty drainage collection bag as each new container is hung and recorded.	

Skill Checklists to Accompany Fundamentals of Nursing:
The Art and Science of Nursing Care, 6th edition

Name _____   Date _____

Unit _____   Position _____

Instructor/Evaluator: _____   Position _____

SKILL 43-8

Applying an External Condom Catheter

Goal: The patient's urinary elimination will be maintained, with a urine output of at least 30 mL/hour, and the bladder is not distended.

Excellent	Satisfactory	Needs Practice		Comments
___	___	___	1. Identify the patient. Discuss procedure with the patient and assess the patient's ability to assist with the procedure. Discuss any allergies with the patient, especially to latex.	
___	___	___	2. Bring the necessary equipment to bedside. Obtain assistance from another staff member, if necessary. Perform hand hygiene. Put on disposable gloves.	
___	___	___	3. Close curtains around bed and close door to room if possible.	
___	___	___	4. Raise the bed to a comfortable working height. Stand on the patient's right side if you are right handed or on the patient's left side if you are left handed.	
___	___	___	5. Prepare urinary drainage setup or reusable leg bag for attachment to condom sheath.	
___	___	___	6. Position the patient on his back with thighs slightly apart. Drape the patient so that only the area around the penis is exposed. Slide waterproof pad under the patient.	
___	___	___	7. Put on disposable gloves. Trim any long pubic hair that is in contact with the penis.	
___	___	___	8. Clean the genital area with washcloth, skin cleanser, and warm water. If the patient is uncircumcised, retract the foreskin and clean glans of penis. Replace the foreskin. Clean the tip of the penis first, moving the washcloth in a circular motion from the meatus outward. Wash the shaft of the penis using downward strokes toward the pubic area. Rinse and dry. Remove gloves. Perform hand hygiene again.	
___	___	___	9. Apply skin protectant to penis and allow to dry.	
___	___	___	10. Roll condom sheath outward onto itself. Grasp penis firmly with nondominant hand. **Apply condom sheath by rolling it onto penis with dominant hand. Leave 1″ to 2″ (2.5 to 5 cm) of space between tip of penis and end of condom sheath.**	
___	___	___	11. Apply pressure to sheath at the base of penis for 10 to 15 seconds.	

Applying an External Condom Catheter *(Continued)*

Excellent	Satisfactory	Needs Practice		Comments
——	——	——	12. Connect condom sheath to drainage setup. Avoid kinking or twisting drainage tubing.	
——	——	——	13. Remove gloves. Secure drainage tubing to the patient's inner thigh with Velcro leg strap or tape. Leave some slack in tubing for leg movement.	
——	——	——	14. Assist the patient to a comfortable position. Cover the patient with bed linens. Place the bed in the lowest position.	
——	——	——	15. Secure drainage bag below the level of the bladder. Check that drainage tubing is not kinked and that movement of side rails does not interfere with the drainage bag.	

Skill Checklists to Accompany Fundamentals of Nursing:
The Art and Science of Nursing Care, 6th edition

Name _____   Date _____

Unit _____   Position _____

Instructor/Evaluator: _____   Position _____

SKILL 43-9

Changing a Stoma Appliance on an Ileal Conduit

Goal: The stoma appliance is applied correctly to the skin to allow urine to drain freely.

Excellent	Satisfactory	Needs Practice		Comments
——	——	——	1. Identify the patient. Explain procedure and encourage the patient to observe or participate if possible.	
——	——	——	2. Perform hand hygiene.	
——	——	——	3. Close curtains around bed and close door to room if possible.	
——	——	——	4. Have the patient sit or stand if able to assist with skill or assume supine position in bed. If in bed, raise the bed to a comfortable working height. Place waterproof pad under the patient at the stoma site.	
——	——	——	5. Place a disposable waterproof pad on the over bed table. Set up the wash basin with warm water and the rest of the supplies. Place a trash bag within reach.	
——	——	——	6. Put on nonsterile gloves. Empty pouch being worn into graduated container if it is not attached to straight drainage.	
——	——	——	7. **Gently remove pouch faceplate from skin by pushing skin from appliance rather than pulling appliance from skin. Start at the top of the appliance, while keeping the abdominal skin taut. If resistance is felt, use warm water or adhesive remover to aid in removal.**	
——	——	——	8. Place the used appliance in the trash bag, if the appliance is a disposable one. If it is a reusable one, set it aside to wash in lukewarm soap and water and allow to air dry after the new appliance is in place.	
——	——	——	9. Clean skin around stoma with mild soap and water or a cleansing agent and a washcloth. Remove all old adhesive from skin; use an adhesive remover if necessary.	
——	——	——	10. Gently pat area dry. **Make sure skin around stoma is thoroughly dry.** Assess stoma and condition of surrounding skin.	
——	——	——	11. Place one or two gauze squares over stoma opening.	
——	——	——	12. Apply skin protectant to a 2″ (5-cm) radius around the stoma, and allow it to dry completely, which takes about 30 seconds.	

SKILL 43-9

Changing a Stoma Appliance on an Ileal Conduit *(Continued)*

Excellent	Satisfactory	Needs Practice		Comments
——	——	——	13. Lift the gauze squares for a moment and measure the stoma opening, using the measurement guide. Replace the gauze. Trace the same size opening on the back center of the appliance. Cut the opening 1/8″ larger than the stoma size.	
——	——	——	14. Remove the backing from the appliance. Quickly remove the gauze squares and discard appropriately; ease the appliance over the stoma. **Gently press onto the skin while smoothing over the surface. Apply gentle pressure to appliance for 5 minutes.**	
——	——	——	15. Secure optional belt to appliance and around patient.	
——	——	——	16. Remove gloves. Assist the patient to a comfortable position. Cover the patient with bed linens. Place the bed in the lowest position.	
——	——	——	17. Put on clean gloves. Remove or discard any remaining equipment and assess the patient's response to procedure. Remove gloves and perform hand hygiene.	

Skill Checklists to Accompany Fundamentals of Nursing:
The Art and Science of Nursing Care, 6th edition

Name _____   Date _____

Unit _____   Position _____

Instructor/Evaluator: _____   Position _____

SKILL 44-1

Administering a Large-Volume Cleansing Enema

Excellent	Satisfactory	Needs Practice	**Goal:** The patient expels feces.	**Comments**
——	——	——	1. Verify the order for the enema. Identify the patient. Explain the procedure to the patient. Discuss where the patient will defecate. Have a bedpan, commode, or nearby bathroom ready for use.	
——	——	——	2. Warm solution in the amount ordered, and check the temperature with a bath thermometer if available. If a bath thermometer is not available, warm to room temperature or slightly higher, and test on inner wrist. If tap water is used, adjust temperature as it flows from the faucet.	
——	——	——	3. Perform hand hygiene.	
——	——	——	4. Add enema solution to the container. Release the clamp and allow fluid to progress through the tube before reclamping.	
——	——	——	5. Pull the curtains around the bed and close the room door. If the bed is adjustable, place it in high position.	
——	——	——	6. Position the patient on the left side (Sims position), as dictated by patient comfort and condition. Fold top linen back just enough to allow access to the patient's rectal area. Place a waterproof pad under the patient's hip.	
——	——	——	7. Put on nonsterile gloves.	
——	——	——	8. Elevate solution so that it is no higher than 18 inches (45 cm) above the level of the anus. Plan to give the solution slowly over a period of 5 to 10 minutes. The container may be hung on an IV pole or held in the nurse's hands at the proper height.	
——	——	——	9. Generously lubricate the end of the rectal tube 2 to 3 inches (5 to 7 cm). A disposable enema set may have a prelubricated rectal tube.	
——	——	——	10. Lift buttock to expose anus. Slowly and gently insert the enema tube 3 to 4 inches (7 to 10 cm) for an adult. Direct it at an angle pointing toward the umbilicus, not bladder. Ask the patient to take several deep breaths.	

Administering a Large-Volume Cleansing Enema (Continued)

Excellent	Satisfactory	Needs Practice		Comments
——	——	——	11. If resistance is met while inserting tube, permit a small amount of solution to enter, withdraw tube slightly, and then continue to insert it. Do not force entry of the tube. Ask the patient to take several deep breaths.	
——	——	——	12. Introduce solution slowly over a period of 5 to 10 minutes. Hold tubing all the time that solution is being instilled.	
——	——	——	13. Clamp tubing or lower container if the patient has the desire to defecate or cramping occurs. The patient also may be instructed to take small, fast breaths or to pant.	
——	——	——	14. After the solution has been given, clamp the tubing and remove the tube. Have a paper towel ready to receive the tube as it is withdrawn.	
——	——	——	15. Return the patient to a comfortable position. Encourage the patient to hold the solution until the urge to defecate is strong, usually in about 5 to 15 minutes. Make sure the linens under the patient are dry. Remove your gloves and ensure that the patient is covered.	
——	——	——	16. Raise the side rail. Lower the bed height and adjust the head of bed to a comfortable position.	
——	——	——	17. Remove any remaining equipment. Perform hand hygiene.	
——	——	——	18. When the patient has a strong urge to defecate, place him or her in a sitting position on a bedpan or assist to a commode or the bathroom. Stay with the patient or have call light readily accessible.	
——	——	——	19. Remind the patient not to flush commode before the nurse inspects the results of the enema.	
——	——	——	20. Put on gloves and assist the patient if necessary with cleaning of the anal area. Offer washcloths, soap, and water for handwashing. Remove gloves.	
——	——	——	21. Leave the patient clean and comfortable. Care for equipment properly.	
——	——	——	22. Perform hand hygiene.	

Skill Checklists to Accompany Fundamentals of Nursing:
The Art and Science of Nursing Care, 6th edition

Name _____   Date _____

Unit _____   Position _____

Instructor/Evaluator: _____   Position _____

SKILL 44-2

Changing and Emptying an Ostomy Appliance

Goal: The stoma appliance is applied correctly to the skin to allow stool to drain freely.

Excellent	Satisfactory	Needs Practice		Comments
___	___	___	1. Gather necessary equipment. Identify the patient. Explain the procedure and encourage the patient to observe or participate if possible.	
___	___	___	2. Close curtains around the bed and close the door to the room if possible.	
___	___	___	3. Perform hand hygiene.	
___	___	___	4. Assist the patient to a comfortable sitting or lying position in bed or a standing or sitting position in the bathroom.	
			Emptying an Appliance	
___	___	___	5. Put on disposable gloves. Remove the clamp and fold the end of pouch upward like a cuff.	
___	___	___	6. Empty contents into a bedpan, toilet, or measuring device. Rinse appliance or pouch with tepid water in a squeeze bottle.	
___	___	___	7. Wipe the lower 2″ of the appliance or pouch with toilet tissue.	
___	___	___	8. Uncuff the edge of the appliance or pouch and apply a clip or clamp. Remove gloves. If the appliance is not to be changed, perform hand hygiene. Assist the patient to a comfortable position.	
			Changing an Appliance	
___	___	___	9. Place a disposable pad on the work surface. Set up the wash basin with warm water and the rest of the supplies. Place a trash bag within reach.	
___	___	___	10. Put on clean gloves. Place a waterproof pad under the patient at the stoma site. Empty the appliance as previously described.	
___	___	___	11. Gently remove pouch faceplate from the skin by pushing skin from the appliance, rather than pulling appliance from skin. Start at the top of the appliance, while keeping the abdominal skin taut. Push the skin from the appliance, rather than pulling the appliance from the skin.	

Excellent	Satisfactory	Needs Practice		Comments
——	——	——	12. Place the appliance in the trash bag, if disposable. If reusable, set it aside to wash in lukewarm soap and water and allow to air dry after the new appliance is in place.	
——	——	——	13. Use toilet tissue to remove any excess stool from the stoma. Cover the stoma with a gauze pad. Clean the skin around the stoma with mild soap and water or a cleansing agent and a washcloth. Remove all old adhesive from the skin; an adhesive remover may be used. Do not apply lotion to the peristomal area.	
——	——	——	14. Gently pat the area dry. Make sure the skin around the stoma is thoroughly dry. Assess the stoma and condition of the surrounding skin.	
——	——	——	15. Apply skin protectant to a 2-inch (5-cm) radius around the stoma, and allow it to dry completely, which takes about 30 seconds.	
——	——	——	16. Lift the gauze squares for a moment and measure the stoma opening, using the measurement guide. Replace the gauze. Trace the same size opening on the back center of the appliance. Cut the opening 1/8 inch larger than the stoma size.	
——	——	——	17. Remove the backing from the appliance. Quickly remove the gauze squares and ease the appliance over the stoma. Gently press onto the skin while smoothing over the surface. Apply gentle pressure to appliance for 5 minutes.	
——	——	——	18. Close the bottom of the appliance or pouch by folding the end upward and using the clamp or clip that comes with the product.	
——	——	——	19. Remove gloves. Assist the patient to a comfortable position. Cover the patient with bed linens. Place the bed in the lowest position.	
——	——	——	20. Put on clean gloves. Remove or discard equipment and assess the patient's response to the procedure. Remove gloves and perform hand hygiene.	

Skill Checklists to Accompany Fundamentals of Nursing:
The Art and Science of Nursing Care, 6th edition

Name _____   Date _____

Unit _____   Position _____

Instructor/Evaluator: _____   Position _____

Excellent	Satisfactory	Needs Practice	SKILL 44-3 **Irrigating a Colostomy**	Comments
			Goal: The patient expels soft formed stool.	
____	____	____	1. Assemble necessary equipment. Verify the order for the irrigation. Identify the patient. Explain the procedure to patient. Plan where he or she will receive the irrigation. Assist the patient onto a bedside commode or into a nearby bathroom.	
____	____	____	2. Pull the curtains around the bed and close the room door. Drape the patient to keep him/her covered.	
____	____	____	3. Warm the solution in the amount ordered, and check the temperature with a bath thermometer if available. If a bath thermometer is not available, warm to room temperature or slightly higher, and test on inner wrist. If tap water is used, adjust temperature as it flows from the faucet.	
____	____	____	4. Perform hand hygiene.	
____	____	____	5. Add irrigation solution to the container. Release the clamp and allow fluid to progress through the tube before reclamping.	
____	____	____	6. Hang the container so that bottom of bag will be at the patient's shoulder level when the patient is seated.	
____	____	____	7. Put on nonsterile gloves.	
____	____	____	8. Remove the ostomy appliance and attach the irrigation sleeve. Place drainage end into the bedpan, toilet bowl, or commode.	
____	____	____	9. Lubricate the end of the cone with water-soluble lubricant.	
____	____	____	10. Insert the cone into the stoma. Introduce solution slowly over a period of 5 to 6 minutes. Hold tubing (or if patient is able, allow patient to hold tubing) all the time that the solution is being instilled. Control the rate of flow by closing or opening the clamp.	
____	____	____	11. **Hold cone in place for an additional 10 seconds after fluid is infused.**	
____	____	____	12. Remove the cone. The patient should remain seated on the toilet or bedside commode.	

Irrigating a Colostomy *(Continued)*

Excellent	Satisfactory	Needs Practice		Comments
____	____	____	13. After the majority of the solution has returned, allow the patient to clip (close) the bottom of the irrigating sleeve and continue with daily activities.	
____	____	____	14. After the solution has stopped flowing from the stoma, put on clean gloves. Remove the irrigating sleeve and cleanse the skin around stoma opening with mild soap and water. Gently pat the peristomal skin dry.	
____	____	____	15. Attach a new appliance to the stoma or stoma cover (see Skill 44-2) as needed.	
____	____	____	16. Remove gloves. Return the patient to a comfortable position. Make sure the linens under the patient are dry, if appropriate. Ensure that the patient is covered.	
____	____	____	17. Raise side rail. Lower bed height and adjust head of bed to a comfortable position.	
____	____	____	18. Perform hand hygiene.	

Skill Checklists to Accompany Fundamentals of Nursing:
The Art and Science of Nursing Care, 6th edition

Name _____   Date _____

Unit _____   Position _____

Instructor/Evaluator: _____   Position _____

Excellent	Satisfactory	Needs Practice	SKILL 45-1 **Using a Pulse Oximeter**	Comments
			Goal: The patient will exhibit arterial blood oxygen saturation within acceptable parameters, or greater than 95%.	
——	——	——	1. Identify the patient using at least two methods.	
——	——	——	2. Explain what you are going to do and why you are going to do it to the patient.	
——	——	——	3. Perform hand hygiene.	
——	——	——	4. Select an adequate site for application of the sensor.	
——	——	——	a. Use the patient's index, middle, or ring finger.	
——	——	——	b. Check the proximal pulse and capillary refill at the pulse closest to the site.	
——	——	——	c. If circulation at site is inadequate, consider using the earlobe or bridge of nose.	
——	——	——	d. Use a toe only if lower extremity circulation is not compromised.	
——	——	——	5. Select proper equipment:	
——	——	——	a. If one finger is too large for the probe, use a smaller one. A pediatric probe may be used for a small adult.	
——	——	——	b. Use probes appropriate for patient's age and size.	
——	——	——	c. Check if patient is allergic to adhesive. A nonadhesive finger clip or reflectance sensor is available.	
——	——	——	6. Prepare the monitoring site. Cleanse the selected area with the alcohol wipe or disposable cleansing cloth. Allow the area to dry. If necessary, remove nail polish and artificial nails after checking manufacturer's instructions.	
——	——	——	7. **Apply probe securely to skin. Make sure that the light-emitting sensor and the light-receiving sensor are aligned opposite each other (not necessary to check if placed on forehead or bridge of nose).**	
——	——	——	8. Connect the sensor probe to the pulse oximeter, turn the oximeter on, and check operation of the equipment (audible beep, fluctuation of bar of light or waveform on face of oximeter).	
——	——	——	9. Set alarms on pulse oximeter. Check manufacturer's alarm limits for high and low pulse rate settings.	

Excellent	Satisfactory	Needs Practice	SKILL 45-1 **Using a Pulse Oximeter** *(Continued)*	
				Comments
——	——	——	10. **Check oxygen saturation at regular intervals, as ordered by physician and signaled by alarms. Monitor hemoglobin level.**	
——	——	——	11. Remove sensor on a regular basis and check for skin irritation or signs of pressure (every 2 hours for spring tension sensor or every 4 hours for adhesive finger or toe sensor).	
——	——	——	12. Clean non-disposable sensors according to the manufacturer's directions. Perform hand hygiene.	

Name _____   Date _____

Unit _____   Position _____

Instructor/Evaluator: _____   Position _____

Excellent	Satisfactory	Needs Practice	SKILL 45-2 **Suctioning the Nasopharyngeal and Oropharyngeal Airways**	Comments
			Goal: The patient will exhibit improved breath sounds and a clear, patent airway.	
___	___	___	1. Identify the patient.	
___	___	___	2. Determine the need for suctioning. Verify the suction order in the patient's chart, if necessary. **For postoperative patient, administer pain medication before suctioning.**	
___	___	___	3. Explain what you are going to do and the reason to the patient, even if the patient does not appear to be alert. Reassure patient you will interrupt procedure if he or she indicates respiratory difficulty.	
___	___	___	4. Perform hand hygiene.	
___	___	___	5. Adjust bed to comfortable working position. Lower side rail closer to you. If patient is conscious, place him or her in a semi-Fowler's position. **If patient is unconscious, place him or her in the lateral position, facing you. Move the bed table close to your work area and raise to waist height.**	
___	___	___	6. Place towel or waterproof pad across patient's chest.	
___	___	___	7. **Adjust suction to appropriate pressure:** For a wall unit for an adult: 100 to 150 mm Hg; neonates: 60 to 80 mm Hg; infants: 80 to 100 mm Hg; children: 100 to 120 mm Hg. For a portable unit for an adult: 10 to 15 cm Hg; neonates: 6 to 8 cm Hg; infants: 8 to 10 cm Hg; children: 10 to 12 cm Hg **Put on a disposable, nonsterile glove and occlude the end of the connecting tubing to check suction pressure. Place the connecting tubing in a convenient location.**	
___	___	___	8. **Open sterile suction package using aseptic technique. The open wrapper or container becomes a sterile field to hold other supplies. Carefully remove the sterile container, touching only the outside surface. Set it up on the work surface and pour sterile saline into it.**	
___	___	___	9. Place a small amount of water-soluble lubricant on the sterile field, taking care to avoid touching the sterile field with the lubricant package.	

Excellent	Satisfactory	Needs Practice	

SKILL 45-2
Suctioning the Nasopharyngeal and Oropharyngeal Airways *(Continued)*

Comments

Excellent	Satisfactory	Needs Practice	
___	___	___	10. Increase the patient's supplemental oxygen level or apply supplemental oxygen per facility policy or physician order.
___	___	___	11. Put on face shield or goggles and mask. Put on sterile gloves. **The dominant hand will manipulate the catheter and must remain sterile. The nondominant hand is considered clean rather than sterile and will control the suction valve (Y port) on the catheter.**
___	___	___	12. With dominant gloved hand, pick up sterile catheter. Pick up the connecting tubing with the nondominant hand and connect the tubing and suction catheter.
___	___	___	13. Moisten the catheter by dipping it into the container of sterile saline. Occlude Y-tube to check suction.
___	___	___	14. Encourage the patient to take several deep breaths.
___	___	___	15. Apply lubricant to the first 2 to 3 inches of the catheter, using the lubricant that was placed on the sterile field.

___	___	___	16. Remove the oxygen delivery device, if appropriate. Do not apply suction as the catheter is inserted. Hold the catheter between your thumb and forefinger.
			    For nasopharyngeal suctioning: **Gently insert catheter through the naris and along the floor of the nostril toward trachea.** Roll the catheter between your fingers to help advance it. Advance the catheter approximately 5 to 6 inches to reach the pharynx.
			    For oropharyngeal suctioning: Insert catheter through the mouth, along the side of the mouth toward the trachea. Advance the catheter 3 to 4 inches to reach the pharynx.

___	___	___	17. Apply suction by intermittently occluding the Y port on the catheter with the thumb of your nondominant hand, and gently rotate the catheter as it is being withdrawn. **Do not suction for more than 10 to 15 seconds at a time.**
___	___	___	18. Replace the oxygen delivery device using your nondominant hand, if appropriate, and have the patient take several deep breaths.
___	___	___	19. Flush catheter with saline. Assess effectiveness of suctioning and repeat as needed and according to patient's tolerance. Wrap the suction catheter around your dominant hand between attempts.

Excellent	Satisfactory	Needs Practice	SKILL 45-2 **Suctioning the Nasopharyngeal and Oropharyngeal Airways** *(Continued)*	
				Comments
——	——	——	20. Allow at least a 30-second to one-minute interval if additional suctioning is needed. No more than three suction passes should be made per suctioning episode. Alternate the nares, unless contraindicated, if repeated suctioning is required. Do not force catheter through the nares. Encourage patient to cough and deep breathe between suctioning. Suction the oropharynx after suctioning the nasopharynx.	
——	——	——	21. When suctioning is completed, remove gloves from dominant hand over the coiled catheter, pulling it off inside out. Remove glove from nondominant hand and dispose of gloves, catheter, and container with solution in the appropriate receptacle. Remove face shield or goggles and mask. Perform hand hygiene.	
——	——	——	22. Turn off suction. Remove supplemental oxygen placed for suctioning, if appropriate. Assist patient to a comfortable position. Raise bed rail.	
——	——	——	23. Offer oral hygiene after suctioning.	
——	——	——	24. Reassess patient's respiratory status, including respiratory rate, effort, oxygen saturation, and lung sounds.	

Skill Checklists to Accompany Fundamentals of Nursing:
The Art and Science of Nursing Care, 6th edition

Name _____ Date _____

Unit _____ Position _____

Instructor/Evaluator: _____ Position _____

Excellent	Satisfactory	Needs Practice	SKILL 45-3 **Administering Oxygen by Nasal Cannula**	Comments
			Goal: The patient will exhibit an oxygen saturation level within acceptable parameters.	
___	___	___	1. Identify the patient using at least two methods.	
___	___	___	2. Explain what you are going to do and the reason to the patient. Review safety precautions necessary when oxygen is in use. Place "no smoking" signs in appropriate areas.	
___	___	___	3. Perform hand hygiene.	
___	___	___	4. **Connect nasal cannula to oxygen setup with humidification, if one is in use.** Adjust flow rate as ordered by physician. Check that oxygen is flowing out of prongs.	
___	___	___	5. Place prongs in patient's nostrils. Place tubing over and behind each ear with adjuster comfortably under chin or around the patient's head, with adjuster at the back of the head or neck. Place gauze pads at ear beneath the tubing as necessary.	
___	___	___	6. Adjust the fit of the cannula as necessary. Tubing should be snug, but not tight against the skin.	
___	___	___	7. **Encourage patient to breathe through the nose, with mouth closed.**	
___	___	___	8. Reassess patient's respiratory status, including respiratory rate, effort, and lung sounds. Note any signs of respiratory distress, such as tachypnea, nasal flaring, use of accessory muscles, or dyspnea.	
___	___	___	9. Perform hand hygiene.	
___	___	___	10. Put on clean gloves. Remove and clean the cannula and assess nares at least every 8 hours, or according to agency recommendations. Check nares for evidence of irritation or bleeding.	

Skill Checklists to Accompany Fundamentals of Nursing:
The Art and Science of Nursing Care, 6th edition

Name _____   Date _____

Unit _____   Position _____

Instructor/Evaluator: _____   Position _____

Excellent	Satisfactory	Needs Practice	SKILL 45-4 **Administering Oxygen by Mask**	
			Goal: The patient exhibits an oxygen saturation level within acceptable parameters.	**Comments**
——	——	——	1. Identify the patient.	
——	——	——	2. Explain what you are going to do and the reason to the patient. Review safety precautions necessary when oxygen is in use. Place "no smoking" signs in appropriate areas.	
——	——	——	3. Perform hand hygiene.	
——	——	——	4. Attach face mask to oxygen source (with humidification, if appropriate for the specific mask). Start the flow of oxygen at the specified rate. For a mask with a reservoir, be sure to allow oxygen to fill the bag before proceeding to the next step.	
——	——	——	5. Position face mask over patient's nose and mouth. Adjust the elastic strap so that the mask fits snugly but comfortably on the face. Adjust the flow rate to the prescribed rate.	
——	——	——	6. If the patient reports irritation or redness is noted, use gauze pads under the elastic strap at pressure points to reduce irritation to ears and scalp.	
——	——	——	7. Reassess patient's respiratory status, including respiratory rate, effort, and lung sounds. Note any signs of respiratory distress, such as tachypnea, nasal flaring, use of accessory muscles, or dyspnea.	
——	——	——	8. Perform hand hygiene.	
——	——	——	9. **Remove the mask and dry the skin every 2 to 3 hours if the oxygen is running continuously. Do not use powder around the mask.**	

Skill Checklists to Accompany Fundamentals of Nursing:
The Art and Science of Nursing Care, 6th edition

Name _____   Date _____

Unit _____   Position _____

Instructor/Evaluator: _____   Position _____

Excellent	Satisfactory	Needs Practice	SKILL 45-5 **Suctioning the Tracheostomy: Open System** **Goal:** The patient will exhibit improved breath sounds and a clear, patent airway.	Comments
___	___	___	1. Identify the patient.	
___	___	___	2. Determine the need for suctioning. Verify the suction order in the patient's chart. **For postoperative patient, administer pain medication as prescribed before suctioning.**	
___	___	___	3. Explain what you are going to do and the reason to the patient, even if the patient does not appear to be alert. Reassure patient you will interrupt procedure if he or she indicates respiratory difficulty.	
___	___	___	4. Perform hand hygiene.	
___	___	___	5. Adjust bed to comfortable working position. Lower side rail closer to you. If patient is conscious, place him or her in a semi-Fowler's position. **If patient is unconscious, place him or her in the lateral position, facing you. Move the over-the-bed table close to your work area and raise to waist height.**	
___	___	___	6. Place towel or waterproof pad across patient's chest.	

___	___	___	7. **Turn suction to appropriate pressure:**
			    For a wall unit for an adult: 100 to 150 mm Hg; neonates: 60 to 80 mm Hg; infants: 80 to 100 mm Hg; children: 100 to 120 mm Hg
			    For a portable unit for an adult: 10 to 15 cm Hg; neonates: 6 to 8 cm Hg; infants 8 to 10 cm Hg; children 10 to 12 cm Hg
			    Put on a disposable, nonsterile glove and occlude the end of the connecting tubing to check suction pressure. Place the connecting tubing in a convenient location. If using it, place resuscitation bag connected to oxygen within convenient reach.	

___	___	___	8. **Open sterile suction package using aseptic technique. The open wrapper or container becomes a sterile field to hold other supplies. Carefully remove the sterile container, touching only the outside surface. Set it up on the work surface and pour sterile saline into it.**	

Excellent	Satisfactory	Needs Practice	SKILL 45-5 **Suctioning the Tracheostomy: Open System** *(Continued)*	Comments
——	——	——	9. Put on face shield or goggles and mask. Put on sterile gloves. **The dominant hand will manipulate the catheter and must remain sterile. The nondominant hand is considered clean rather than sterile and will control the suction valve (Y port) on the catheter.**	
——	——	——	10. With dominant gloved hand, pick up sterile catheter. Pick up the connecting tubing with the nondominant hand and connect the tubing and suction catheter.	
——	——	——	11. Moisten the catheter by dipping it into the container of sterile saline, unless it is a silicone catheter. Occlude Y-tube to check suction.	
——	——	——	12. Using your nondominant hand and a manual resuscitation bag, hyperventilate the patient delivering three to six breaths or use the sigh mechanism on a mechanical ventilator.	
——	——	——	13. Open the adapter on the mechanical ventilator tubing or remove oxygen delivery setup with your nondominant hand.	
——	——	——	14. Using your dominant hand, gently and quickly insert catheter into trachea. **Advance the catheter to the predetermined length. Do not occlude Y-port when inserting catheter.**	
——	——	——	15. Apply suction by intermittently occluding the Y port on the catheter with the thumb of your nondominant hand, and gently rotate the catheter as it is being withdrawn. **Do not suction for more than 10 to 15 seconds at a time.**	
——	——	——	16. Hyperventilate the patient using your nondominant hand and a manual resuscitation bag, delivering 3 to 6 breaths. Replace the oxygen delivery device, if applicable, using your nondominant hand and have the patient take several deep breaths. If the patient is mechanically ventilated, close the adapter on the mechanical ventilator tubing and use the sigh mechanism on a mechanical ventilator.	
——	——	——	17. Flush catheter with saline. Assess effectiveness of suctioning and repeat as needed and according to patient's tolerance. Wrap the suction catheter around your dominant hand between attempts.	

Excellent	Satisfactory	Needs Practice		Comments
___	___	___	18. Allow at least a 30-second to one-minute interval if additional suctioning is needed. No more than three suction passes should be made per suctioning episode. Encourage patient to cough and deep breathe between suctionings. Suction the oropharynx after suctioning the trachea. Do not reinsert in the tracheostomy after suctioning the mouth.	
___	___	___	19. When suctioning is completed, remove gloves from dominant hand over the coiled catheter, pulling it off inside out. Remove glove from nondominant hand and dispose of gloves, catheter, and container with solution in the appropriate receptacle. Remove face shield or goggles and mask. Perform hand hygiene.	
___	___	___	20. Turn off suction. Assist patient to a comfortable position. Raise bed rail. Offer oral hygiene after suctioning.	
___	___	___	21. Reassess patient's respiratory status, including respiratory rate, effort, oxygen saturation, and lung sounds.	

Skill Checklists to Accompany Fundamentals of Nursing:
The Art and Science of Nursing Care, 6th edition

Name _____ Date _____

Unit _____ Position _____

Instructor/Evaluator: _____ Position _____

Excellent	Satisfactory	Needs Practice	SKILL 45-6 **Providing Tracheostomy Care**	Comments
			Goal: The patient will exhibit a tracheostomy tube and site free from drainage, secretions, and skin irritation or breakdown.	
——	——	——	1. Identify the patient.	
——	——	——	2. Determine the need for tracheostomy care. **Assess patient's pain and administer pain medication, if indicated.**	
——	——	——	3. Explain what you are going to do and the reason to the patient, even if the patient does not appear to be alert. Reassure patient you will interrupt procedure if he or she indicates respiratory difficulty.	
——	——	——	4. Perform hand hygiene.	
——	——	——	5. Adjust bed to comfortable working position. Lower side rail closer to you. If patient is conscious, place him or her in a semi-Fowler's position. **If patient is unconscious, place him or her in the lateral position, facing you. Move the bed table close to your work area and raise to waist height. Place a trash receptacle within easy reach of work area.**	
——	——	——	6. Put on face shield or goggles and mask. Suction tracheostomy if necessary. If tracheostomy has just been suctioned, remove soiled site dressing and discard prior to removal of gloves used to perform suctioning.	
			Cleaning the Tracheostomy (Nondisposable Inner Cannula)	
——	——	——	7. Prepare supplies:	
——	——	——	a. Open tracheostomy care kit and separate basins, touching only the edges. If kit is not available, open three sterile basins.	
——	——	——	b. Fill one basin 0.5" deep with hydrogen peroxide or $\frac{1}{2}$ hydrogen peroxide and $\frac{1}{2}$ saline, based on facility policy.	
——	——	——	c. Fill other two basins 0.5" deep with saline.	
——	——	——	d. Open sterile brush or pipe cleaners if they are not already available in a cleaning kit. Open additional sterile gauze pad.	
——	——	——	8. Put on disposable gloves.	

SKILL 45-6

Providing Tracheostomy Care *(Continued)*

Excellent	Satisfactory	Needs Practice		Comments

—— —— ——	9.	Remove the oxygen source if one is present. If not already removed, remove site dressing and dispose of in the trash. Stabilize the outer cannula and faceplate of the tracheostomy with one hand. Rotate the lock on the inner cannula in a counterclockwise motion with your other hand to release it.	
—— —— ——	10.	Continue to hold the faceplate. Gently remove the inner cannula and carefully drop it in the basin with hydrogen peroxide. Replace the oxygen source over the outer cannula. Remove gloves and discard.	
—— —— ——	11.	Clean the inner cannula as follows:	
—— —— ——		a. Put on sterile gloves.	
—— —— ——		b. Remove inner cannula from soaking solution. Moisten brush or pipe cleaners in saline and insert into tube, using back-and-forth motion.	
—— —— ——		c. Agitate cannula in saline solution. Remove and tap against inner surface of basin.	
—— —— ——		d. Place on sterile gauze pad.	
—— —— ——	12.	**Suction outer cannula using sterile technique if necessary.**	
—— —— ——	13.	Stabilize the outer cannula and faceplate with one hand. Replace inner cannula into outer cannula. Turn lock clockwise and check that inner cannula is secure. Reapply oxygen source if needed.	

Applying Clean Dressing and Ties/Tape

—— —— ——	14.	Remove oxygen source. Dip cotton-tipped applicator or gauze sponge in second basin with sterile saline and clean stoma under faceplate. **Use each applicator or sponge only once, moving from stoma site outward.**	
—— —— ——	15.	Pat skin gently with dry 4″ × 4″ gauze sponge.	
—— —— ——	16.	Slide commercially prepared tracheostomy dressing or prefolded non-cotton-filled 4″ × 4″ dressing under faceplate.	
—— —— ——	17.	Change the tracheostomy tape:	
—— —— ——		a. **Leave soiled tape in place until new one is applied.**	
—— —— ——		b. Cut piece of tape the length of twice the neck circumference plus 4″. Trim ends of tape on the diagonal.	
—— —— ——		c. Insert one end of tape through faceplate opening alongside old tape. Pull through until both ends are even length.	

Excellent	Satisfactory	Needs Practice		Comments

d. Slide both ends of the tape under patient's neck and insert one end through remaining opening on other side of faceplate. Pull snugly and tie ends in double square knot. You should be able to fit one finger between the neck and the ties. Check to make sure that the patient can flex neck comfortably.

e. Carefully remove old tape. Reapply oxygen source if necessary.

18. Remove face shield or mask and goggles. Remove gloves and discard. Perform hand hygiene. Reassess patient's respiratory status, including respiratory rate, effort, oxygen saturation, and lung sounds.

Skill Checklists to Accompany Fundamentals of Nursing:
The Art and Science of Nursing Care, 6th edition

Name _____ Date _____

Unit _____ Position _____

Instructor/Evaluator: _____ Position _____

Excellent	Satisfactory	Needs Practice	SKILL 46-1 **Starting an Intravenous Infusion**	
			Goal: The IV catheter is inserted using sterile technique on the first attempt. Also, the patient experiences minimal trauma and the IV solution flows freely.	**Comments**
____	____	____	1. Verify the IV order against the physician order. Clarify any inconsistencies. Check the patient's chart for allergies. Check for color, clarity, expiration date, etc.	
____	____	____	2. Know the techniques for IV insertion, precautions, purpose of the IV administration and medications if ordered.	
____	____	____	3. Gather all equipment and bring to the bedside.	
____	____	____	4. Identify the patient. Ask the patient if he/she is allergic to any medication, iodine, or tape, as appropriate. If considering using an anesthetic (numbing) cream or 1% lidocaine injection, check for allergies for these substances as well.	
____	____	____	5. Explain the need for the IV and procedure to the patient.	
____	____	____	6. Perform hand hygiene. If using an anesthetic cream, apply the anesthetic cream to a few potential insertion sites.	
____	____	____	7. Prepare IV solution and tubing:	
____	____	____	a. **Maintain strict aseptic technique when opening sterile packages and IV solution.**	
			b. Clamp IV tubing, uncap spike on the administration set, and insert into the entry site on the IV bag or bottle as the manufacturer directs.	
____	____	____	c. Squeeze the drip chamber and allow it to fill at least halfway.	
____	____	____	d. Remove the cap at end of the IV tubing and while maintaining its sterility, open the IV tubing clamp, and allow fluid to move through tubing. **Allow fluid to flow until all air bubbles have disappeared and the entire length of the tubing is primed (filled) with IV solution.** Close the clamp and recap the end of tubing, maintaining sterility of the setup.	
____	____	____	e. If an electronic device is to be used, follow the manufacturer's instructions for inserting the tubing and setting the infusion rate.	

Excellent	Satisfactory	Needs Practice	SKILL 46-1 **Starting an Intravenous Infusion** *(Continued)*	
				Comments
—	—	—	f. Apply the label if medication was added to container (pharmacy may have added medication and applied the label). Label the tubing with the date and time that tubing was hung.	
—	—	—	g. Place time-tape on the container and hang the IV on the pole.	
—	—	—	8. Place the patient in low Fowler's position in bed. Place protective towel or pad under the patient's arm. Close the door to the room or pull the bedside curtain.	
—	—	—	9. Provide emotional support as needed.	
—	—	—	10. **Select and palpate for an appropriate vein. Avoid an arm that has been compromised, such as with the presence of arteriovenous fistula.**	
—	—	—	11. If the site is hairy and agency policy permits, clip a 2-inch area around the intended site of entry.	
—	—	—	12. Apply a tourniquet 3 to 4 inches above the venipuncture site to obstruct venous blood flow and distend the vein. Direct the ends of the tourniquet away from the site of entry. Make sure the radial pulse is still present.	
—	—	—	13. Instruct the patient to hold the arm lower than the heart.	
—	—	—	14. Ask the patient to open and close the fist. Observe and palpate for a suitable vein. Try the following techniques if a vein cannot be felt:	
—	—	—	a. Massage the patient's arm from proximal to distal end and gently tap over the intended vein.	
—	—	—	b. Remove the tourniquet and place warm moist compresses over the intended vein for 10 to 15 minutes.	
—	—	—	15. Put on clean gloves.	
—	—	—	16. If using intradermal lidocaine, cleanse the insertion site with alcohol using a circular motion. Inject a small amount (0.2 to 0.3 mL) of lidocaine into the area. If numbing cream was used, wipe cream off the insertion site. **Cleanse the site with an antiseptic solution such as chlorhexidine or according to agency policy. Use a circular motion to move from the center outward for several inches.**	
—	—	—	17. Use the nondominant hand, placed about 1 or 2 inches below the entry site, to hold the skin taut against the vein. **Avoid touching the prepared site.** Ask the patient to remain still while the venipuncture is performed.	

Excellent	Satisfactory	Needs Practice	SKILL 46-1 **Starting an Intravenous Infusion** *(Continued)*	Comments
___	___	___	18. Enter the skin gently, holding the catheter by the hub in your dominant hand, bevel side up, at a 10- to 15-degree angle. The catheter may be inserted from directly over the vein or the side of the vein. While following the course of the vein, advance the needle or catheter into the vein. A sensation of "give" can be felt when the needle enters the vein.	
___	___	___	19. When blood returns through the lumen of the needle or the flashback chamber of the catheter, advance either device 1/8 to 1/4 inch farther into the vein. A catheter needs to be advanced until the hub is at the venipuncture site, but the exact technique depends on the type of device used.	
___	___	___	20. Release the tourniquet as soon as possible. Quickly remove the protective cap from the IV tubing and attach the tubing to the catheter or needle. Stabilize the catheter or needle with your nondominant hand.	
___	___	___	21. Start the flow of solution promptly by releasing the clamp on the tubing. Examine the tissue around the entry site for signs of infiltration.	
___	___	___	22. Secure the catheter with narrow nonallergenic tape (1/2 inch) placed with the sticky side up under the hub and crossed over the top of the hub.	
___	___	___	23. **Place sterile dressing over the venipuncture site.** Agency policy may direct nurse to use gauze dressing or transparent dressing. Apply tape to dressing if necessary. Loop the tubing near the site of entry, and anchor to dressing.	
___	___	___	24. Label the IV dressing with the date, time, site, and type and size of catheter used for the infusion on the tape anchoring the tubing.	
___	___	___	25. Remove all equipment and dispose of properly. Remove gloves and perform hand hygiene.	
___	___	___	26. Anchor arm to an armboard for support if necessary, or apply a site protector or tube-shaped mesh netting over the insertion site. Explain to the patient the purpose of the armboard and the importance of safeguarding the site when using the extremity.	
___	___	___	27. Adjust the rate of solution flow according to the amount prescribed, or follow manufacturer's directions for adjusting flow rate on infusion pump.	

Excellent	Satisfactory	Needs Practice	SKILL 46-1 **Starting an Intravenous Infusion** *(Continued)*	Comments
——	——	——	28. Document the procedure and the patient's response. Chart the time, site, device used, and solution.	
——	——	——	29. Return to check the flow rate and observe the IV site for infiltration 30 minutes after starting the infusion. Ask the patient if he/she is experiencing any pain or discomfort related to the IV infusion.	

Skill Checklists to Accompany Fundamentals of Nursing:
The Art and Science of Nursing Care, 6th edition

Name _____   Date _____

Unit _____   Position _____

Instructor/Evaluator: _____   Position _____

Excellent	Satisfactory	Needs Practice	SKILL 46-2 **Changing IV Solution Container and Tubing**	Comments
			Goal: The patient experiences minimal to no trauma when solution and tubing are changed.	
____	____	____	1. Identify the patient. Ask the patient if he/she is allergic to any medication, iodine, or tape, as appropriate.	
____	____	____	2. Gather all equipment and bring to the bedside. Check the IV solution and medication additives against the physician's order. Label the IV if medication is added. Include the date, time, and your name or initials.	
____	____	____	3. Explain the procedure and reason for change to the patient.	
____	____	____	4. Perform hand hygiene.	
			To Change IV Solution Container	
____	____	____	5. Carefully remove protective cover from new IV solution container and expose the bag entry site.	
____	____	____	6. **Close the clamp on the IV tubing. If using an electronic device, turn the device to the "hold" position.**	
____	____	____	7. Lift the container off the IV pole and invert it. **Quickly remove the spike from the old IV container, being careful not to contaminate it.**	
____	____	____	8. Steady the new container and insert the spike. Hang on the IV pole.	
____	____	____	9. Reopen the clamp, check the drip chamber of the administration set on the tubing, and adjust the flow. Readjust the electronic device by turning the device "ON" and verify the programmed flow rate. Inspect for air bubbles in the tubing. If using an electronic device, check that the device is operating correctly.	
____	____	____	10. Label the container according to agency policy. Record on the intake and output record and document on the chart according to agency policy. Discard used equipment properly. Perform hand hygiene.	
			To Change IV Solution Container and Tubing	
____	____	____	11. Prepare the IV solution and tubing, checking the IV order with the physician's order and labeling the IV with the date, time, and name or initials.	

SKILL 46-2

Changing IV Solution Container and Tubing *(Continued)*

Excellent	Satisfactory	Needs Practice		Comments
——	——	——	a. **Maintain strict aseptic technique when opening sterile packages and the IV solution.**	
——	——	——	b. Clamp the IV tubing, uncap the spike on the administration set and insert into the entry site on the IV bag or bottle as the manufacturer directs.	
——	——	——	c. Squeeze the drip chamber and allow it to fill at least halfway.	
——	——	——	d. Remove the cap at end of the IV tubing and while maintaining its sterility, open the IV tubing clamp, and allow fluid to move through the tubing. **Allow fluid to flow until all air bubbles have disappeared** and the entire length of the tubing is primed (filled) with IV solution. Close the clamp and recap the end of the tubing, maintaining sterility of the setup.	
——	——	——	e. If an electronic device is to be used, follow the manufacturer's instructions for inserting the tubing and setting the infusion rate.	
——	——	——	f. Label the tubing with the date and time that tubing was hung.	
——	——	——	g. Place time-tape on the container and hang the IV on the pole.	
——	——	——	12. Close the clamp on the existing IV tubing. Also, close the clamp on the short extension tubing connected to the IV catheter in the patient's arm.	
——	——	——	13. Remove the current infusion tubing from the resealable cap on the short extension IV tubing. Using an antimicrobial wipe, swab the resealable cap and insert the new IV tubing into the cap.	
——	——	——	14. Open the clamp on the IV tubing and on the short extension tubing. Check the IV flow. Readjust the electronic device as needed.	
——	——	——	15. **Regulate the IV flow according to the physician's order.**	
——	——	——	16. **Label the IV tubing with the date, time, and your initials. Label the IV solution container and record the procedure according to agency policy.** Discard used equipment properly and perform hand hygiene.	
——	——	——	17. Record the patient's response to the IV infusion.	

Skill Checklists to Accompany Fundamentals of Nursing:
The Art and Science of Nursing Care, 6th edition

Name _____   Date _____

Unit _____   Position _____

Instructor/Evaluator: _____   Position _____

Excellent	Satisfactory	Needs Practice	SKILL 46-3 **Monitoring an IV Site and Infusion**	Comments
			Goal: The patient remains free from complications and demonstrates signs and symptoms of fluid balance.	
___	___	___	1. Identify the patient.	
___	___	___	2. Monitor the IV infusion every hour or per agency policy. More frequent checks may be necessary if medication is being infused.	
___	___	___	a. Check the physician's order for the IV solution.	
___	___	___	b. Check the drip chamber and time drops if the IV is not regulated by an infusion control device.	
___	___	___	c. Check the tubing for anything that might interfere with flow. Be sure that the clamp is in the open position. Observe dressing for leakage of the IV solution.	
___	___	___	d. Observe settings, alarm, and indicator lights on the infusion control device if one is being used. Educate the patient related to alarm features on the electronic infusion device.	
___	___	___	3. Inspect the site for swelling, leakage at the site, coolness, or pallor, which may indicate infiltration. Ask the patient if he/she is experiencing any pain or discomfort. If so, the IV must be removed and restarted at another site. Check agency policy for treating infiltration.	
___	___	___	4. Inspect the site for redness, swelling, and heat. Palpate for induration. Ask the patient if he/she is experiencing pain. These findings may indicate phlebitis. The IV will need to be discontinued and restarted at another site. Notify the physician if you suspect phlebitis. Check agency policy for treatment of phlebitis.	
___	___	___	5. Check for local (redness, pus, warmth, induration, and pain) that may indicate an infection is present at the site or systemic manifestations (chills, fever, tachycardia, hypotension) that may accompany local infection at the site. The IV should be discontinued and the physician notified. Be careful not to disconnect the IV tubing when putting on the patient's hospital gown.	

Excellent	Satisfactory	Needs Practice	SKILL 46-3 **Monitoring an IV Site and Infusion** *(Continued)*	
				Comments
——	——	——	6. Be alert for additional complications of IV therapy.	
——	——	——	a. **Fluid overload can result in signs of cardiac and/or respiratory failure. Monitor intake and output and vital signs. Assess for edema and auscultate lung sounds. Ask if the patient is experiencing any shortness of breath.**	
——	——	——	b. Bleeding at the site is most likely to occur when the IV is discontinued.	
——	——	——	7. **If possible, instruct the patient to call for assistance if any discomfort is noted at the site, the solution container is nearly empty, the flow has changed in any way, or if the electronic pump alarm sounds.**	

Skill Checklists to Accompany Fundamentals of Nursing:
The Art and Science of Nursing Care, 6th edition

Name _____ Date _____

Unit _____ Position _____

Instructor/Evaluator: _____ Position _____

Excellent	Satisfactory	Needs Practice	SKILL 46-4 **Changing a Peripheral IV Dressing** **Goal:** The patient will exhibit an IV site that is clean, dry, and without evidence of any signs and symptoms of infection, infiltration, or phlebitis.	Comments
——	——	——	1. Identify the patient. Ask the patient if he/she is allergic to any medication, iodine, or tape, as appropriate.	
——	——	——	2. Explain the need for the IV and the procedure to the patient.	
——	——	——	3. **Perform hand hygiene. Put on clean gloves.**	
——	——	——	4. Place a towel or disposable pad under the arm with the IV site. **Carefully remove the old dressing, but leave the tape that anchors the IV needle or catheter in place.** Discard properly.	
——	——	——	5. **Inspect the IV site for the presence of phlebitis (inflammation), infection, or infiltration. If noted, discontinue and relocate IV.**	
——	——	——	6. Loosen and gently remove the tape, being careful to steady the catheter with one hand. Use adhesive remover if necessary.	
——	——	——	7. **Cleanse the entry site with a chlorhexidine solution using a circular motion, moving from the center outward. Allow to dry.**	
——	——	——	8. Reapply tape strip to the needle or catheter at the entry site.	
——	——	——	9. Apply transparent polyurethane dressing over the entry site. Remove gloves and perform hand hygiene.	
——	——	——	10. **Secure the IV tubing with additional tape if necessary. Label dressing with the date, time of change, and your initials. Check that the IV flow is accurate and the system is patent.**	
——	——	——	11. Discard equipment properly and perform hand hygiene.	
——	——	——	12. Record the patient's response to the dressing change and observation of the site.	

Skill Checklists to Accompany Fundamentals of Nursing:
The Art and Science of Nursing Care, 6th edition

Name _____   Date _____

Unit _____   Position _____

Instructor/Evaluator: _____   Position _____

SKILL 46-5

Capping a Primary Line for Intermittent Use

Goal: The patient will remain free of injury and any signs and symptoms of IV complications.

Excellent	Satisfactory	Needs Practice		Comments
____	____	____	1. Gather equipment and verify the physician's order. Fill the syringe with normal saline or heparin flush according to agency policy. Recap the syringe for use in Action 8.	
____	____	____	2. Identify the patient.	
____	____	____	3. Explain the procedure to the patient.	
____	____	____	4. Perform hand hygiene.	
____	____	____	5. Assess the IV site.	
____	____	____	6. **Clamp off the primary IV tubing.**	
____	____	____	7. Put on clean gloves according to hospital policy. Clamp the extension tubing if a clamp is present. Remove the primary IV tubing from the extension set or adapter device. Cleanse the adapter device with an antimicrobial swab.	
____	____	____	8. Unclamp the extension set and insert a saline or heparin flush syringe into the cap. Instill the solution over 1 minute or flush the line according to agency policy. Reclamp the extension tubing and remove the syringe.	
____	____	____	9. Remove gloves and dispose of them appropriately.	
____	____	____	10. Tape the adapter device (and extension tubing if used).	
____	____	____	11. Perform hand hygiene and ensure the patient is comfortable.	
____	____	____	12. Chart on the IV administration record, MAR, or CMAR per institutional policy.	

Skill Checklists to Accompany Fundamentals of Nursing:
The Art and Science of Nursing Care, 6th edition

Name _____   Date _____

Unit _____   Position _____

Instructor/Evaluator: _____   Position _____

Excellent	Satisfactory	Needs Practice	SKILL 46-6 **Administering a Blood Transfusion**	
			Goal: The patient receives the blood transfusion without any evidence of a transfusion reaction or complication.	**Comments**
___	___	___	1. Identify the patient. Ask the patient if he/she is allergic to any medication, iodine, tape or if he/she has had a transfusion or transfusion reaction in the past.	
___	___	___	2. Determine whether the patient knows the reason for the blood transfusion. Explain to the patient what will happen. Check for signed consent for the transfusion if required by agency. Advise the patient to report any chills, itching, rash, or unusual symptoms. If the physician has ordered any premedication, administer it now.	
___	___	___	3. Perform hand hygiene and put on clean gloves.	
___	___	___	4. **Hang container of 0.9% normal saline with blood administration set to initiate IV infusion and follow administration of blood.**	
___	___	___	5. Start the IV with 18 or 19 gauge catheter if not already present (see Skill 46-1). Keep the IV open by starting the flow of normal saline.	
___	___	___	6. Obtain blood product from the blood bank according to agency policy. Scan for bar codes on blood products if required.	
___	___	___	7. **Complete identification and checks as required by agency: identification number; blood group and type; expiration date; patient's name; inspect blood for clots.**	
___	___	___	8. **Take a baseline set of vital signs before beginning the transfusion.**	
___	___	___	9. Start infusion of the blood product:	
___	___	___	a. Prime in-line filter with blood.	
___	___	___	b. **Start the administration slowly (no more than 25 to 50 mL for the first 15 minutes). Stay with the patient for the first 5 to 15 minutes of transfusion.**	
___	___	___	c. **Check vital signs at least every 15 minutes for the first half hour. Follow the institution's recommendations for taking vital signs during the remainder of the transfusion.**	

Excellent | Satisfactory | Needs Practice

Comments

d. Observe patient for flushing, dyspnea, itching, hives, or rash or any unusual comments.

e. Never warm blood in a microwave. Use a blood warming device, if indicated or ordered, especially with rapid transfusions through a CVP catheter.

10. Maintain the prescribed flow rate as ordered or as deemed appropriate based on the patient's overall condition, keeping in mind the outer limits for safe administration. Ongoing monitoring is crucial throughout the entire duration of the blood transfusion for early identification of any adverse reactions. **Assess frequently for transfusion reaction. Stop the blood transfusion if you suspect a reaction. Quickly replace the blood tubing with new tubing and 0.9% sodium chloride. Notify the physician and blood bank.**

11. When the transfusion is complete, clamp off blood and begin to infuse 0.9% normal saline.

12. Record the administration of blood and the patient's reaction as ordered by agency. Return the blood transfusion bag to the blood bank according to agency policy.